Reproduction

Reproduction:

The Cycle of Life

By Karen Jensen and the
Editors of U.S.News Books

U.S.NEWS BOOKS   Washington, D.C.

U.S.NEWS BOOKS

THE HUMAN BODY
Reproduction:
The Cycle of Life

Editor/Publisher: Roy B. Pinchot

Series Editor: Judith Gersten

Picture Editor: Leah Bendavid-Val

Art Director: Jack Lanza

Design Consultant: David M. Seager

Staff Writers
Christopher West Davis
Kathy E. Goldberg
Karen Jensen
Michael Kitch
Charles R. Miller
Doug M. Podolsky
Matthew J. Schudel
Robert D. Selim
Edward O. Welles, Jr.

Director of Text Research: William Rust

Chief Researcher: Bruce A. Lewenstein

Text Researchers
Susana Barañano, Barbara L. Buchman,
Heléne Goldberg, Michael C. McCarthy,
Patricia Madigan, E. Cameron Ritchie,
Ann S. Rosoff, Loraine S. Suskind

Chief Picture Researcher: Jean Shapiro Cantú

Picture Researchers
Ronald M. Davis, Gregory A. Johnson,
Leora Kahn, David Ross, Lynne Russillo,
JoAnn Tooley, Arthur Whitmore

Technical Illustration Layout
Esperance Shatarah

Art Staff
Raymond J. Ferry, Martha Anne Scheele

Director of Production: Harold F. Chevalier

Production Coordinator: Diane B. Freed

Production Assistant: Mary Ann Haas

Production Staff
Carol Bashara, Ina Bloomberg,
Barbara M. Clark, Glenna Mickelson,
Sharon Turner

Quality Control Director: Joseph Postilion

Director of Sales: James Brady

Business Planning: Robert Licht

Fulfillment Director: Debra Hasday Fanshel

Fulfillment Assistant: Diane Childress

Cover Design: Moonink Communications

Cover Art: Paul Giovanopoulos

Series Consultants

Donald M. Engelman is Molecular Biophysicist and Biochemist at Yale University and a guest Biophysicist at the Brookhaven National Laboratory in New York. A specialist in biological structure, Dr. Engelman has published research in American and European journals. From 1976 to 1980, he was chairman of the Molecular Biology Study Section at the National Institutes of Health.

Stanley Joel Reiser is Associate Professor of Medical History at Harvard Medical School and codirector of the Kennedy Interfaculty Program in Medical Ethics at the University. He is the author of *Medicine and the Reign of Technology* and coeditor of *Ethics in Medicine: Historical Perspectives and Contemporary Concerns.*

Harold C. Slavkin, Professor of Biochemistry at the University of Southern California, directs the Graduate Program in Craniofacial Biology and also serves as Chief of the Laboratory for Developmental Biology in the University's Gerontology Center. His research on the genetic basis of congenital defects of the head and neck has been widely published.

Lewis Thomas is Chancellor of the Memorial Sloan-Kettering Cancer Center in New York City. A member of the National Academy of Sciences, Dr. Thomas has served on advisory councils of the National Institutes of Health. He has written *The Medusa and the Snail* and *The Lives of a Cell,* which received the 1974 National Book Award in Arts and Letters.

Consultants for Reproduction

Clifford Grobstein is professor of biological science and public policy at the University of California, San Diego. He has conducted embryological research for several decades in association with the National Cancer Institute, Stanford University and the University of California at San Diego. He is a member of many medical and scientific societies including the National Academy of Sciences and the Institute of Medicine. In 1959, Dr. Grobstein received the Brachet award from the Royal Academy of Sciences in Belgium for his work in embryological research. His most recent book is *From Chance to Purpose: An Appraisal of External Human Fertilization.*

Howard and **Georgeanna Jones** are professors in obstetrics and gynecology and codirectors of the In Vitro Fertilization Program at Norfolk's Eastern Virginia Medical School. The husband-and-wife physicians supervised the birth of Elizabeth Jordan Carr, America's first test-tube baby, in December 1981. The Joneses taught gynecology and obstetrics for more than forty years at Johns Hopkins University School of Medicine in Baltimore, Maryland. They are members of the American Society of Human Genetics and the American Fertility Society.

Sherman J. Silber is a urologist, microsurgeon and specialist in fertility and reproduction at St. Luke's West Medical Center in St. Louis, Missouri. He has developed many scientific innovations in the treatment of infertility, among them the microsurgical reversal of vasectomies and tubal ligations. He performed the first successful testicle transplant in 1977. A writer of medical textbooks on microsurgery and on the prostate, Dr. Silber is also author of *How To Get Pregnant* and *The Male: From Infancy to Old Age.*

Picture Consultants

Amram Cohen is General Surgery Resident at the Walter Reed Army Medical Center in Washington, D.C.

Richard G. Kessel, Professor of Zoology at the University of Iowa, studies cells, tissues and organs with scanning and transmission electron microscopy instruments. He is coauthor of two books on electron microscopy.

U.S.News Books, a division of U.S.News & World Report, Inc.

Copyright © MCMLXXXII
by U.S.News & World Report, Inc.
All rights reserved.
No part of this book may be reproduced in any form or by any means, either electronic or mechanical, including photocopying, recording, or by any information storage and retrieval system, without permission in writing from the publisher.

Library of Congress Cataloging in Publication Data

Jensen, Karen, 1957-
    Reproduction: the cycle of life.

    (The Human body)
    Includes index.
    1. Human reproduction.   I. U.S.News
                                    Books.
II. Title.   III. Series.
QP251.J46   612'.6   82-2745
                                    AACR2
ISBN 0-89193-606-8
ISBN 0-89193-636-X (leatherbound)
ISBN 0-89193-666-1 (school ed.)

20 19 18 17 16 15 14 13 12 11
10   9   8   7   6   5   4   3   2   1

Contents

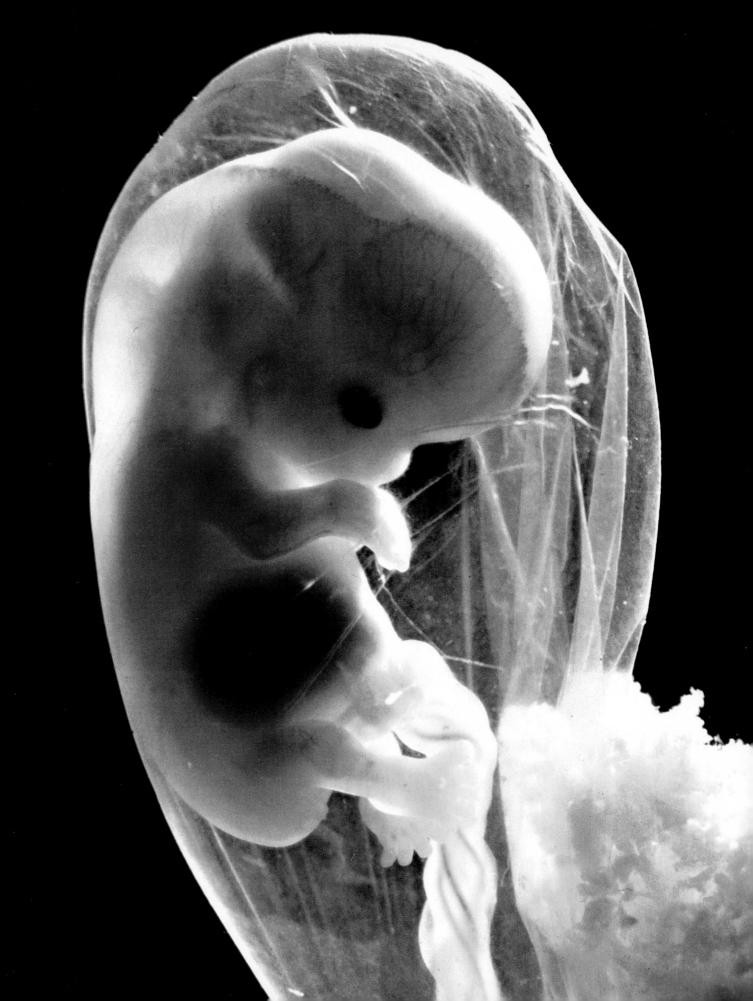

Introduction:

Replenishing Our Kind

From its microscopic origin, an embryo blooms into human form, weaving a new thread of its history with every turn it takes. Heeding unspoken commands, cells grow active, moving with busy purpose to create a new life and endow it with sense, feeling and movement. A fetus steadily acquires vigor and insensibly refines the functions of life that will endure from the protected world of the womb through experience and age.

A newborn baby gasps for air with its first cry, filling lungs that have never breathed before. It opens its eyes and peers out on an unfamiliar world. If capable of speech, it could recite the odyssey of its own birth, a tale worthy of poets. William Wordsworth must have thought of this extraordinary journey when he wrote:

> Not in entire forgetfulness
> And not in utter nakedness,
> But trailing clouds of glory do we come.

The lore of procreation — part fact, part fiction — has long dictated the ways we approach pregnancy and birth. The story of reproduction fascinates us as much as it did our forebears who fashioned totems of fertility for spiritual benefit. Through science, some of the mysteries surrounding birth have been shed, but new puzzles have been unveiled. Still, even the scientists who have altered traditional notions of reproduction stand in amazement at the forces that mingle together as life.

Man is indeed a fruitful animal. Our numbers attest to our success in filling the biological niche that our ancestors carved. The chronicle of reproduction, though, is more than a study of biology. Perhaps more than any other natural act of man, it engages emotions and the imagination. Birth is universally celebrated as an occasion of joy and as an event that unites families in a shared bond. With its initial breath, a child spreads hope and embodies a spirit of the future.

Enwrapped by a gauze of membrane, a baby journeys unseen for nine months, undergoing such changes and growth as will never occur again. Alone in the womb, he could almost, like Hamlet, count himself "a king of infinite space." An unborn baby is the soul of helplessness but also, as blood begins to flow in his veins, a symbol of continuity and of aspirations fulfilled.

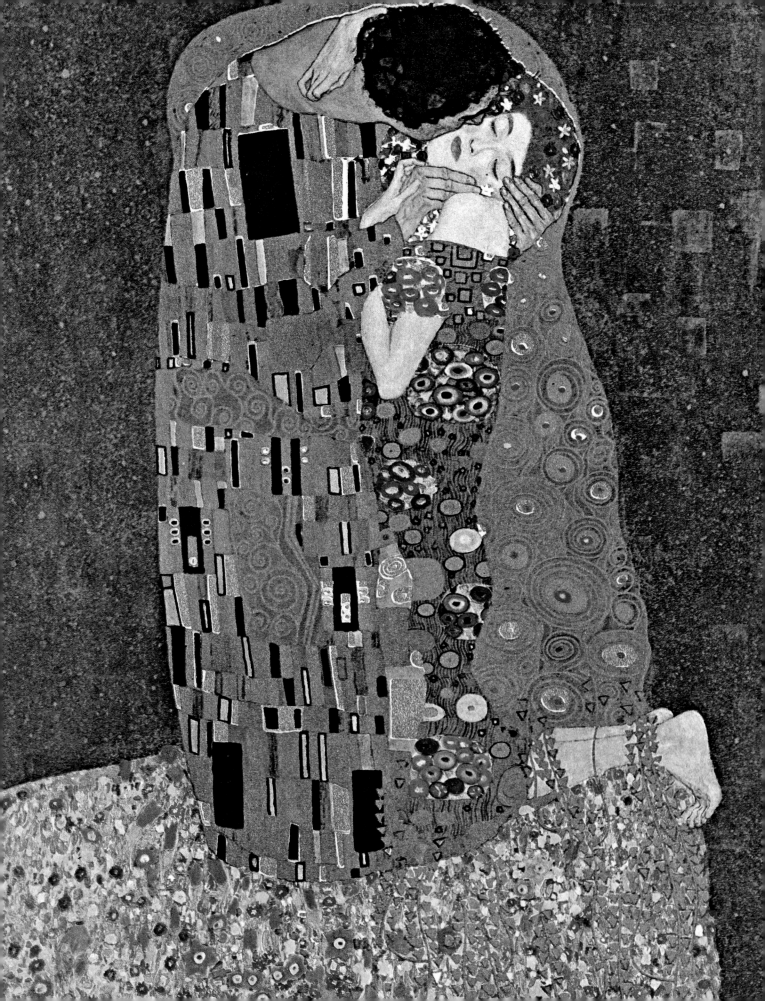

Chapter 1

From Genesis to Genetics

Entwined in a timeless embrace, the shimmering lovers in Gustav Klimt's The Kiss *embody the mystery that engenders life and legend. Since earliest times, mankind has sought to discover the origin of new life. From genesis to genetics, we have come far.*

Through the ages, a curtain of superstition and ignorance veiled the mystery of conception. In the millennia before man gained a fundamental understanding of fertilization and genetics, people of all cultures created myths to explain the entrance of new generations into the world. From earliest times, birds and other creatures were endowed through folklore with the means to foster life. Ancient Hindus and Egyptians attributed the power of genesis to gods, aided by flocks of ibises that guarded their masters' powers. The ancients prayed to the ibis, believing it carried babies to those whom the gods favored.

The stork, a relative of the ibis, inspired perhaps the most enduring myth of human reproduction. Faith in the stork's procreative powers originated with the Teutons, an ancient Celtic people who lived across much of what is now northern Europe. In secret swamps and ponds, feeding grounds of these long-legged birds, the souls of unborn children were thought to dwell. There the storks gathered up spirit children and ferried them to people's homes. The birds' habit of returning to the same nesting places every year made them omens of good fortune and fertility. The Teutons believed that couples who wished to have no children had simply to shoo the stork away. Even in years when the stork's visits and the birth of a child did not correspond, Teutons clung to their myth, rationalizing unwanted pregnancies by assuming that the stork had somehow eluded their vigilance and slipped in to deliver a child under the cover of darkness.

The stork myth found believers in England, Germany, Scandinavia and elsewhere in Europe. In many households, the birds were thought to be not only bearers of children, but their fathers as well — sometimes impregnating a woman simply by flying above the house. Some husbands built stork shelters on roofs in the hope of attracting the awkward birds, thereby blessing their marriage with many children. Parents who wished to have larger families assigned their first-born child to sprinkle sugar on windowsills to bait a stork. Even after people's faith in the powers of the stork waned, the legend lived on. Parents told inquiring children that storks sometimes bit a mother's leg while bringing babies, appeasing for the moment, at least, children's natural curiosity about birth and conveniently explaining why expectant mothers needed bed rest before a baby's arrival.

The Spirit Children

Other legends explaining pregnancy told of spirit children whose souls inhabited the fruit of trees and the waters of rivers, pools and streams. Women of southern Melanesia believed they risked pregnancy by eating fruit that harbored the spirits' souls. With its symbolic ties to birth and the womb, immersion in water commonly appeared in pregnancy myths. Women bathing in streams were warned to avoid the eyes of crabs watching by the water's edge. Papuans thought fish, eels, water snakes and other phallic creatures awaited the chance to impregnate women who ventured into deep waters. Some anthropologists say these legends originated with primitive tribes, who, finding no connection between the sex act and pregnancy, thought all babies came from the spirit world. Among Australian aborigines and other primitive societies, a young girl's early experiences with sexual intercourse would often begin years before she was biologically able to conceive children. When she eventually conceived, sexual intercourse and the birth of a child nine months later would not necessarily seem related. Instead, the sun, wind, rain and especially the moon and stars were often associated with fertility and conception. Even in modern times, some childless women of northwestern India stand naked before the warm rays of the sun to invoke its fertile powers.

Although the process of human conception remained a mystery to some cultures, other ancient civilizations were keenly aware that new life has its origin in the union of male and female. In the prehistoric cave dwellings of Tuc d'Audoubert,

This eighteenth-century woodcut depicts an age-old myth of South Pacific islanders. In Melanesian society, pregnancy was bestowed upon women who ate fruit harboring the souls of spirit children. The human fruit grows amid the foliage. Fluttering their wings in the tree's shade stand birdlike figures, fertility symbols in conception myths dating back to the ancient Egyptians.

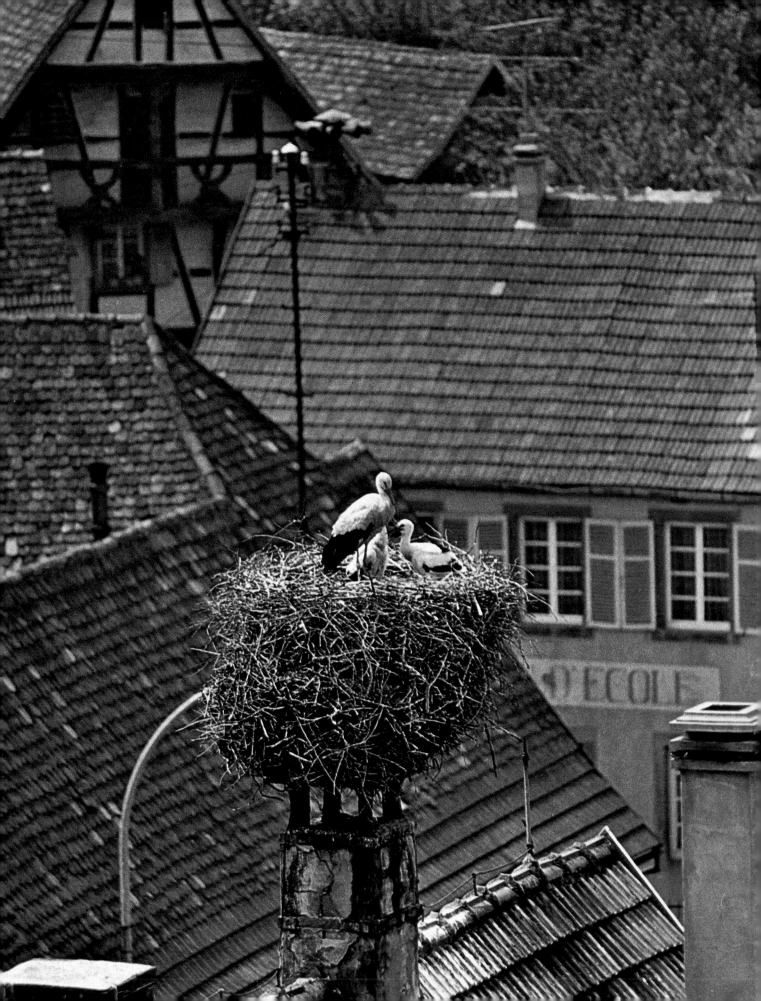

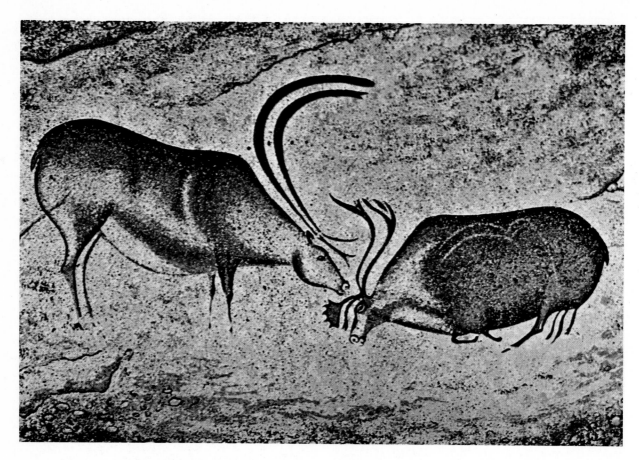

Cave-dwelling hunters drew fertility scenes during magic rituals to ensure a large herd. The cave painting found in Font de Gaume, France, above, depicts a male deer nuzzling a female while she gives birth. The fragment of a clay tablet from the ancient civilization of Phoenicia, right, reveals at least a rudimentary understanding of the importance of the union of man and woman for procreation. The emphasis on the woman's lactating breast and the man's penis shows a rough knowledge of sexual physiology. But the palm trees, serpents, sun and fish underscore the mystery that has surrounded reproduction since earliest times.

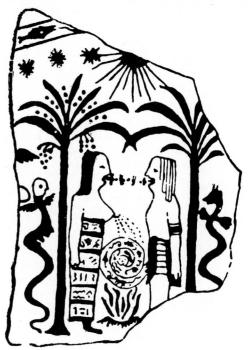

France, archaeologists unearthed phallic models of clay, tributes to man's procreative power. Wall paintings of bison in sexual union, apparently part of fertility rituals, were probably the creations of hunters seeking to assure large herds. In China, yin and yang, male and female, are the two great principles that rule the universe. In Hindu cultures, the power of Shiva and Shakti, the male and female gods, permeates all life.

Many ancient cultures crafted statues, amulets and paintings of sexual organs as tokens of fertility for both womb and field. Some authorities think these images were idolized even before man worshipped gods. In magic rites, believers used symbols of male and female reproductive organs to cajole supernatural powers into warding off evil spirits and bestowing the blessings of fecundity. An ancient Japanese legend tells of Mitoshi-no-Kami, the god of rice, who dispatched a swarm of locusts in an outburst of rage to ruin a village's rice crop. Seeking to pacify the god, the farmers offered him a wooden figure with a huge phallus. Among some Japanese farmers, the practice continues today. Such offerings and rites were intended to encourage fertility and abundance during the seasonal labors of plowing, sowing and harvesting. Through rituals which often included sexual intercourse, peasants around the world sought to earn the favor of the gods of fertility. Remnants of the rituals persisted for hundreds of years. To the end of the nineteenth century in Europe, some peasants still joined sexually with their wives in the fields to promote a good harvest.

Ancient Greeks depended upon statues of the phallus and vulva, separately and in union, to protect them from the evil eye and other spirits, whose ominous presence could bring misfortune to household and village. Images of genitals were thought to break evil spells. Exposing the vulva, especially of a menstruating woman, was thought to have a magic effect against bad weather, hard times and malevolent spells.

Where sorcery and superstition abounded, pregnant women and newborn children were believed to be endangered by the magic of evil wishers. Shakespeare's Caliban, the malformed and brutish slave in *The Tempest*, is a mooncalf.

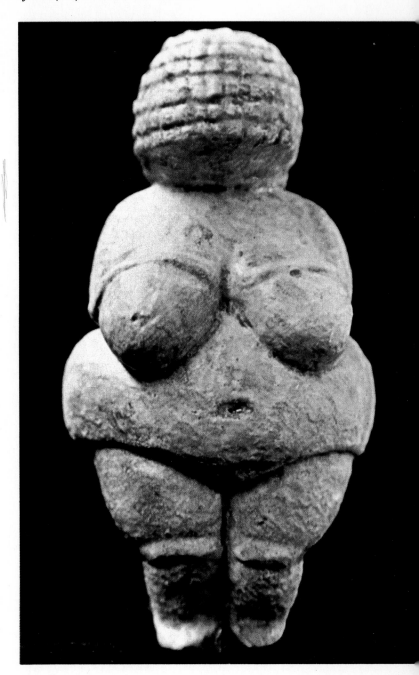

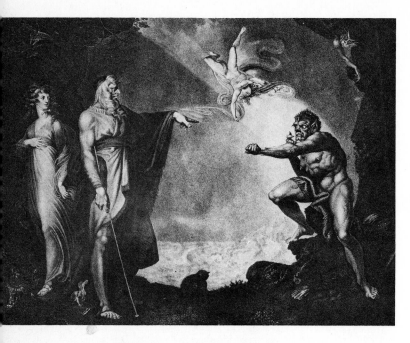

Caliban, the grotesquely mis-shapen slave in Shakespeare's The Tempest, *was a mooncalf, an unborn child transformed into a mythical monster when the moon cast her evil eye upon his mother.*

The creature was so named from an ancient belief that the eye of the moon could cast a spell upon expectant mothers, transforming their unborn children into grotesque monsters. The bridal veil may originally have served to protect brides from the evil eye, which might otherwise doom first-born children to an early grave.

Birth Magic

Ancient Teutonic tribes considered difficult labor to be proof of a woman's infidelity. Likewise, frail or dark babies were thought to be "changelings," fairies that nymphs left in the cradle in exchange for an infant. The Celts believed the changeling, a very old spirit, could only be destroyed if tricked into revealing its true age. In the Scottish Highlands, the suspected changeling would be held above a peat fire to force the fairy from the baby's body. Many ancient cultures also regarded multiple births with foreboding. In the Congo, superstition forced the separation of twins from other members of the tribe and deemed all articles used by twins taboo. The unusualness of the birth of twins was regarded as proof of their unearthliness. To this day in northwest India, a woman who dies within ten days of giving birth is said to become Hedali, an especially threatening spirit.

Myths of benevolence also surrounded the mysteries of birth. As late as the nineteenth century in England, some people believed that a child born with a caul, part of a torn fetal membrane adhering to a child's head, possessed positive magical powers. Whoever possessed the "holy hood," as it was sometimes called, gained the power of second sight. Sailors in particular prized cauls as protection against drowning. One of Charles Dickens's most famous characters, David Copperfield, was born with a caul, "which was advertised for sale, in the newspapers, at the low price of fifteen guineas."

In some parts of the world, the placenta and umbilical cord were valued as cures for barrenness and impotence. People in cultures that believed these relics of birth were the seat of the child's soul observed unusual precautions in disposing of them. The Kwakiutl Indians of British Columbia cast a boy's placenta to ravens, hoping

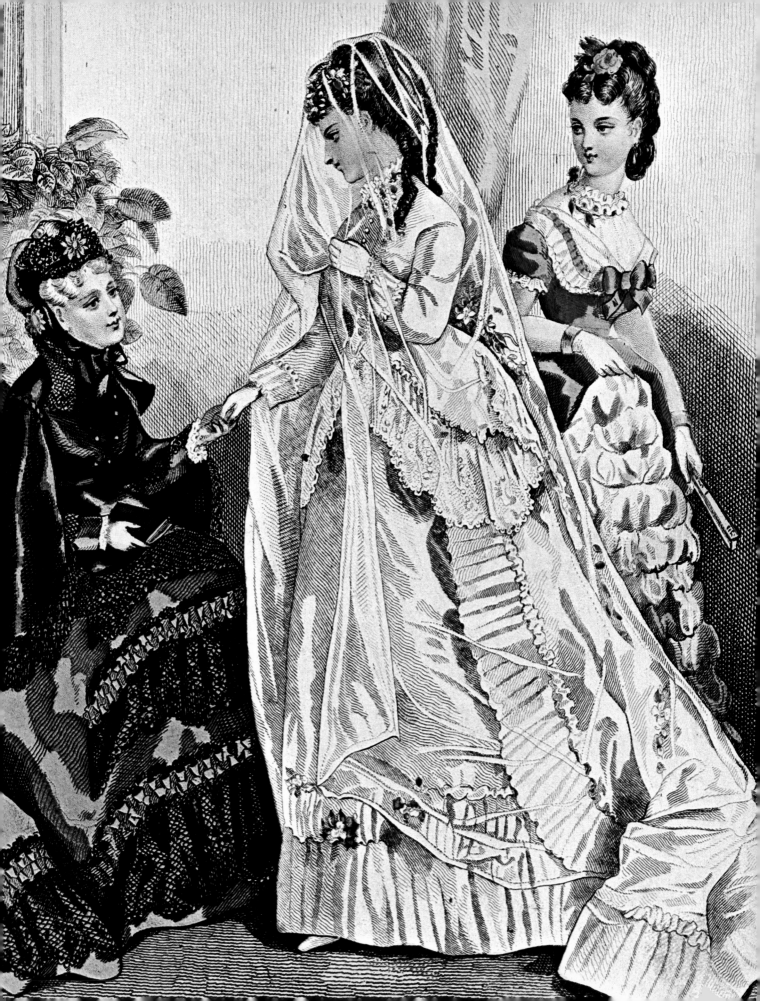

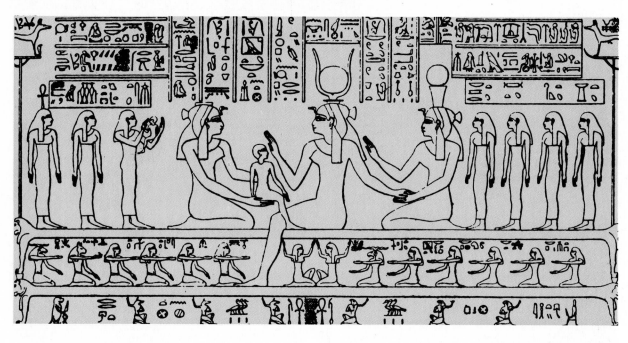

to bestow upon him the power to see into the future. A girl's placenta was buried near the sea at the high-tide line so that she would become a good clam digger.

Science and Superstition

Side by side with such fanciful notions arose a medical interest in pregnancy and birth, first set down in Egyptian hieroglyphics around 2000 B.C. Translations of Egyptian papyri, which include the earliest known gynecological writings, reveal a surprising mixture of superstition and brilliant observation. This combination was the reflection of a remarkably sophisticated society in which physicians diagnosed the internal origins of maladies for the first time. Though some of the prescriptions now seem based on naive concepts, the Egyptians were aware of the link between intercourse and pregnancy as well as some biological causes of female infertility. To determine pregnancy, one papyrus recommended watering wheat and barleycorns with a patient's urine. If the plants grew rapidly, pregnancy was confirmed. Modern scientists have tested this assay and found it to be 80 percent accurate. The particular combination of hormones present only in the urine of pregnant women affects the growth of the plants. The same ancient physicians, however, regarded the uterus as an independent animal that could change form and even wander throughout the body. In diagnosing abdominal pains, physicians conducted external and vaginal examinations to determine the uterus's position and the temporary animal form it had taken. Sometimes it was tortoise-shaped and at other times assumed the form of a newt or crocodile. Egyptian religious beliefs, prohibiting dissections, may have led to such meager familiarity with female reproductive anatomy. "To determine who will bear and who will not bear: you should place an onion bulb deep in her flesh leaving it there all night until dawn," one papyrus advised. "If the odor of it appears in her mouth she will give birth, if it does not she will never give birth."

Progress in understanding conception was slow. Fifteen hundred years later in Greece, the great physician Hippocrates recommended the same sort of procedure. "If a woman does not conceive and you wish to ascertain whether she can," Hippocrates prescribed wrapping her in blankets and fumigating her lower body. "If it appears that the odor passes through her body to the nostrils, and to the mouth, know that of herself she is not unfruitful." If that didn't work, physicians could turn to another method, which required that a woman drink a brew containing human milk and watermelon. Subsequent vomiting was held as a sure sign of fertility but simple belching meant the woman was infertile.

Seed and Soil

Hippocrates, too, mixed misconceptions with insight. He maintained that semen existed both in men and women, but he correctly argued that both sexes contributed to the formation of a child. His theory was controversial for the time. Never before had a physician suggested that a woman was more than the soil in which a man planted his seed. Hippocrates thought semen was "separated from every part of the body, from the solid parts as well as from the soft parts and from every fluid that is in the body." He also believed that in the semen of both man and woman there was a female element and a male element. "If after intercourse, the woman is not going to conceive, the semen from both usually passes out at her will. If, on the other hand, she is going to conceive, the semen does not pass out but stays in the womb . . . and a mixture is effected of that which comes from the man and that which comes from the woman." Hippocrates concluded that the male element in semen was stronger than the female element. If both sexes contributed the stronger element of their semen to conception, a male was born, and the combination of the weaker elements produced a female. The same man and woman did not always supply strong or weak semen, but different semen at different times. After conception occurred, Hippocrates surmised, menstrual blood somehow flowed up into the womb to form the flesh of the offspring.

Aristotle, born in Hippocrates' last years of life, strongly opposed all notions of a female contribution to the creation of offspring. He conceded the importance of menstrual blood, but only as nourishment for the developing fetus. "The mother of what is called a child is no parent," Aristotle declared, "but only a nurse to the young life that is sown in her. The parent is the male — she is only a stranger, a friend whose fate bears the plant, preserving it until it is put forth."

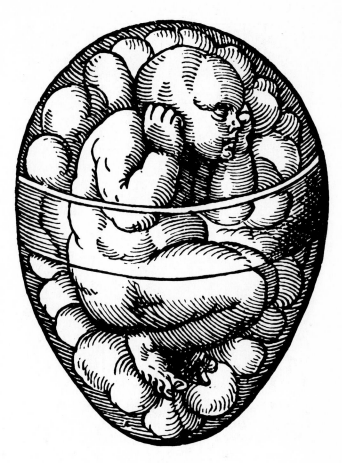

To Aristotle, the mother was only "a nurse to the young life that is sown in her." This sixteenth-century woodcut illustrates the ancient view that a human mother's role was strictly to incubate the offspring, but depicts the embryo inside an egg. That mammals also have a kind of egg, the ovum, was not discovered until the nineteenth century.

17

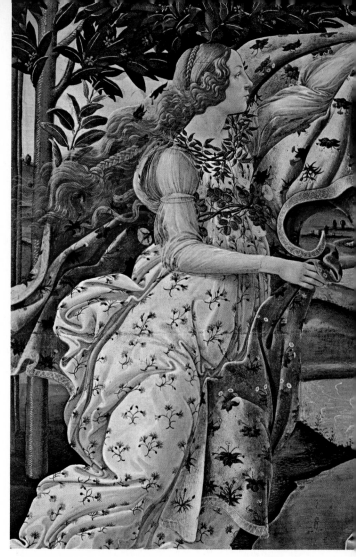

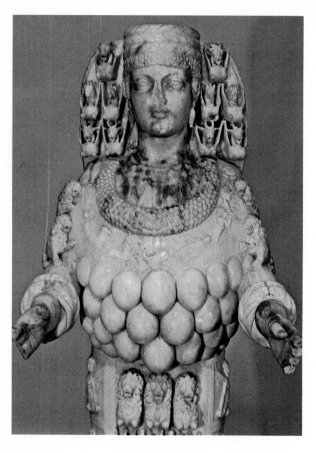

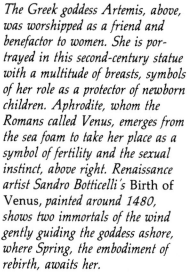

The Greek goddess Artemis, above, was worshipped as a friend and benefactor to women. She is portrayed in this second-century statue with a multitude of breasts, symbols of her role as a protector of newborn children. Aphrodite, whom the Romans called Venus, emerges from the sea foam to take her place as a symbol of fertility and the sexual instinct, above right. Renaissance artist Sandro Botticelli's Birth of Venus, *painted around 1480, shows two immortals of the wind gently guiding the goddess ashore, where Spring, the embodiment of rebirth, awaits her.*

Contesting Hippocratic theory, Aristotle declared that semen entered the woman's body to ignite a series of dynamic forces that formed the offspring. Semen had only an "intrinsic vital heat — a heat that has nothing to do with fire." Males developed in the left side of the womb, which was warmer, and females on the right. The movement of the winds, he reasoned, also affected the semen's vital heat. More males were born under northern winds, and females, southern.

The Life Force

The sexual urge was a transcendent creative force to the ancient Greeks, and around it sprang up rituals, gods and cults. Aphrodite, born of sea foam, was the goddess of love. A symbol of fertility as well as the sexual instinct, she was the celestial generative force and her influence pervaded all nature. Cults arose worshipping her as both the guardian of marriage and the goddess of

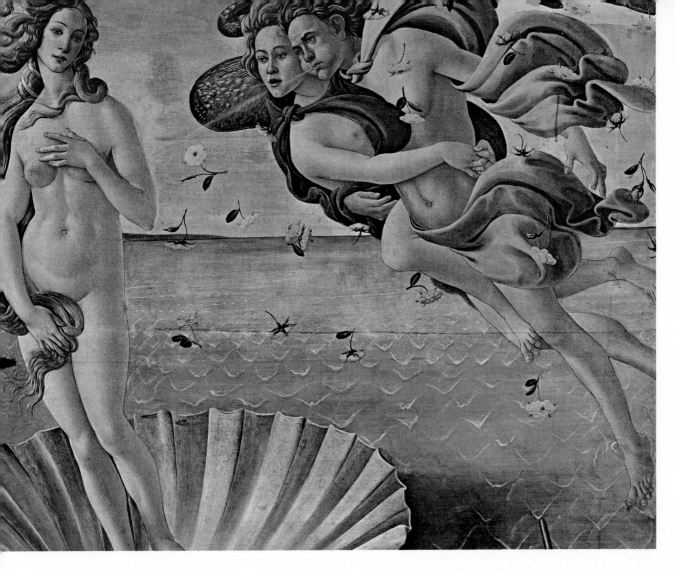

whores. At Corinth, worshippers performed rites of sacred prostitution in her name. Artemis, goddess of childbirth, granted fertility to man and beast. Friend to woman, Artemis was portrayed with a multitude of breasts, symbolizing her maternal role as a protector of infants and children.

Some cults preached that the sexual union of devotee with priest or priestess, who symbolized the worshipped deity, sometimes led to exaltation. One such cult surrounded Zeus, king of gods and men, and his wife Hera. In ceremonies performed for centuries in Greece, mortal couples sought a fleeting expansion of consciousness that transformed the sexual into the celestial.

Later, Romans worshipped Priapus, whose symbol was an erect phallus. During temple celebrations, an enormous phallus carved of cypress and adorned with flowers was carried in procession. Followers of Priapus would fasten symbols of the male and female genitals to the statue in the hope that the god would bless them with abundant fertility. Traditionally, brides would enter the garden of Priapus's temple before marriage. There, the bride was led to the phallus of Priapus's statue to sacrifice her virginity in order to attain his supreme blessings. As Rome degenerated into moral decay, the worship of Priapus grew and the god became the embodiment of sexual and material pleasures.

Amid the debauchery of Rome, a Greek physician, Soranus of Ephesus, developed new concepts of gynecology and obstetrics. Using a crude vaginal speculum to peer into the vagina, he was the first to accurately describe common uterine movements. The womb seemed to wander, observed Soranus, "not because it is animal-like, as some believe, but because . . . it has sensitiveness" to the contractions of uterine ligaments. Refuting Aristotle, he accepted the importance of the woman's role in conception and heredity.

Fathering Obstetrics

Like many physicians of his era, Soranus of Ephesus, a Greek, was eventually drawn to Rome. Born in Asia Minor in the first century A.D., he journeyed to Alexandria, Egypt, the intellectual center of the Mediterranean, to learn the art of medicine. From there, Soranus traveled to the city of seven hills, where he practiced his profession during the rule of the emperors Trajan and Hadrian.

Soranus belonged to the methodist sect of medicine, a school holding that some mysterious constriction and relaxation of the body's "internal pores" dictated sickness and well-being. But Soranus's brilliance as a physician more than overcame his flaws as a physiologist. *Gynecology*, his collection of treatises on midwifery and women's diseases, reflected the practice of ancient obstetrical and gynecological medicine at its finest.

Soranus wrote in an age when faith in miracle cures by the gods was waning. His work helped usher in a new rationalism. Marked most by their objectivity, his writings reveal his contempt for the Roman worship of medical deities. "The midwife should be no believer in spirits," Soranus scolded. She "must be literate," he said, "in order to be

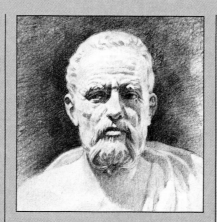

able to comprehend the art through theory, too."

However skeptical of contemporary magical beliefs Soranus was, he did assume the existence of a "natural sympathy" between the uterus and breasts. But even where he lacked scientific evidence, his instincts were right. Modern knowledge of hormones and the nervous system vindicates Soranus's belief in a kind of physiological "sympathy."

Gynecology, written for physicians, midwives and laymen, described abnormal and normal events that might occur during pregnancy and birth. It included advice for midwives and a short account of the female reproductive system. The work concluded with the proper ways of swaddling, bathing, massaging and weaning infants as well as treatment of childhood diseases.

Soranus's insight into the process of giving birth brought a previously unknown comfort to the laboring mother. "One must first soothe the pains by touching with warm hands, and afterwards drench pieces of cloth with warm, sweet olive oil and put them over the abdomen," he prescribed. "There should be three woman helpers, capable of gently allaying the [pregnant woman's] anxiety." He disdained drugs that hastened labor and physicians who applied force to hurry birth. For fetuses positioned transversely in the womb, Soranus reintroduced a method of delivery that entailed gently turning the fetus so that it would emerge feet first, in the breech position. Still risky, a breech birth gave the child at least a chance of survival. His method is used today in hospitals worldwide.

Soranus died in the second century A.D., soon after the birth of Galen, another Greek physician who rose to fame in Rome. Galen, whose influence would dominate medicine for centuries, ridiculed methodist teachings, but never those of Soranus. The Middle Ages accepted Soranus's writings as dogma. And in the age of scientific creativity that followed, they became the cornerstone of gynecology and obstetrics.

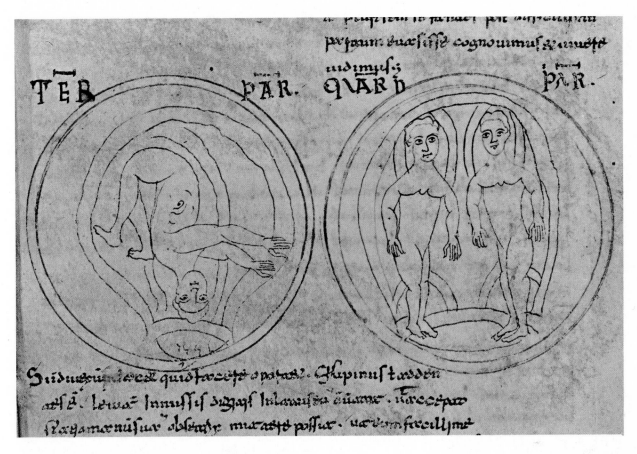

Soranus's contemporary Claudius Galenus, known to history as Galen, also believed that women played some vital role in conception, although he could not muster the scientific evidence. Believing semen was a derivative of blood, Galen concluded that the coagulation of male and female semen in the uterus formed the membranous foundation of the embryo. Nevertheless, it was generally accepted that only men served an active role in generation. This particular misconception and a broader ignorance of the facts of human reproduction allowed superstition to reign unchallenged for the next thousand years.

The Renaissance, when intellectual and artistic achievement once again flourished, brought an end to many age-old fallacies concerning reproduction. Leonardo da Vinci, the great Italian artist and engineer, at first accepted Aristotle's theory that the woman's role in procreation was solely to provide nourishment for the offspring.

The thousand years of the Middle Ages interrupted medical progress. When learned men again explored the causes of human maladies, they turned to ancient texts. This twelfth-century manuscript based on the teachings of Soranus, who had lived a thousand years earlier, shows fetal positions that complicate pregnancies. The umbilical cords are missing, however, revealing that the drawings are somewhat unfaithful to Soranus's writings.

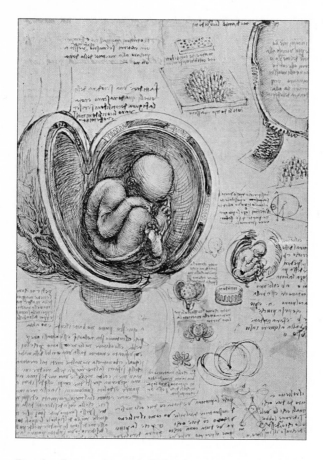

canal, he speculated, that the soul or "animal spirit" was conducted during coition from the man to the future embryo. Early drawings of the uterus presented paired tubes, one of which extended upward to the mammary glands, the milk-producing organs in the female breast. The sketches were probably an attempt to integrate the ancient notion that menstrual blood, retained during pregnancy, passed through this vessel to be changed into milk by the breasts. The second vessel was thought to carry blood to the ovary, where it was converted into female sperm. These initial attempts to represent the uterus showed two distinct chambers within the organ, the prevailing view from ancient times. But a note on one of Leonardo's illustrated parchments reveals his discontent with his early drawings. "I have wasted my hours," he wrote. In his later figures, he drew the uterus as a single chamber. Leonardo clearly drew the urethral orifice but neglected the external female reproductive organs. Fifty years would pass before an Italian anatomist would accurately describe them.

That man was Gabriello Fallopio. Familiar with the texts of Hippocrates, Galen and other ancient physicians, in 1561 Fallopio published his own *Observationes Anatomicae*. He provided elegant interpretations of human anatomy punctuated with theories of function and comparative anatomy. Fallopio was the first to recognize that connective tissue was an element of muscle. He also identified and delineated parts of the vascular and autonomic nervous systems as well as much of the anatomy of the inner ear. But his greatest contribution was his study of female anatomy. He did as much as any scientist to sweep away the ignorance surrounding women's reproductive organs. Dissecting cadavers, Fallopio studied the clitoris, the female erectile organ, and the hymen, the membrane occluding the vaginal opening. He gave scientific names to the vagina and placenta and his notes suggest that he observed hormonal glands as well as various ligaments and muscles in the reproductive tract. Fallopio is best known for his discovery of the pair of slender ducts connecting the uterus to the ovaries — the Fallopian tubes. He came across them while searching for the origin of female semen so often mentioned in

But he later adopted Galen's views, saying that the fetus was "always fashioned out of the two seeds." Sketching internal anatomy during dissections, he depicted the body's structure with unprecedented grace and preciseness. Most of his anatomical drawings were lost until the end of the eighteenth century. Had they been available to scientists in Leonardo's time, a sound understanding of human anatomy might not have been so long in coming. Still, Leonardo misinterpreted what he saw. While many of his depictions were accurate to the finest detail, his drawings of the male and female reproductive organs seem today an odd combination of accuracy and distortion.

In sketching the dissected penis, Leonardo drew two internal canals. The lower one, the urethra, served to conduct sperm and urine from the body. The top canal, perhaps nothing more than a superficial vein, was drawn as though it were connected to the spinal cord. It was through this

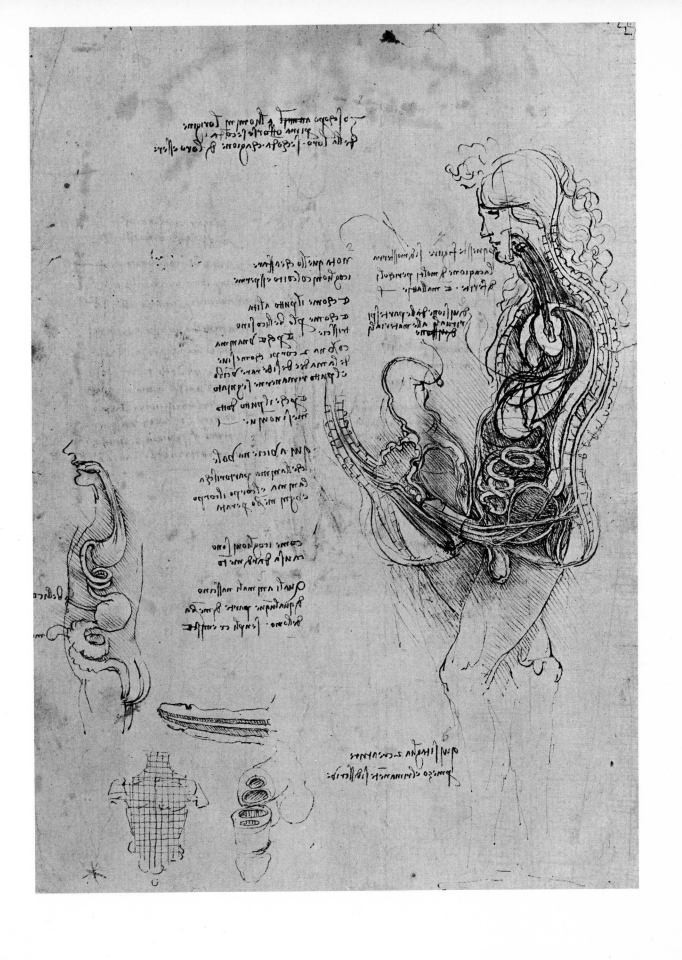

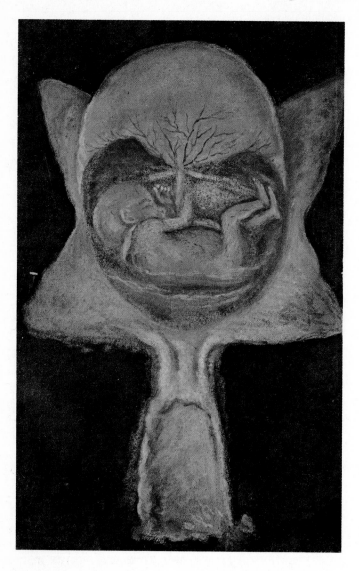

Hieronymus Fabricius, the anatomist who laid the foundations of embryology, illustrated his theories. His painting of a fetus inside the womb, below, combines beauty and accuracy. Fabricius was the first scientist to accurately describe and paint the placenta, opposite page. The membranous organ lines the uterine wall and gathers food and oxygen which are carried to the fetus through the umbilical cord.

the ancient texts. The tubes, Fallopio wrote, resembled "the tendrils of a vine." Upon opening them, he compared their internal structure to "the bell-like mouth of a bronze trumpet."

One of Fallopio's students at Italy's renowned University of Padua was Hieronymus Fabricius. Emulating his mentor's career, Fabricius practiced medicine and surgery while perfecting his skills as an anatomist. His book, *The Formed Fetus,* published in 1600, described the embryonic development of man and various animals, paying special attention to the structural changes in the vascular systems of women after childbirth. Fabricius proposed the revolutionary concept that the egg was the germ from which every animal took shape — even those thought to arise spontaneously. He theorized that male seminal fluid interacted somehow with the female egg, but the specifics eluded him. It would be another two centuries before a scientist would discover that mammals have internal eggs, or ova.

William Harvey, famed seventeenth-century English physician, agreed with the concept *omnia ex ovo* — that all life comes from the egg. He believed that the ovum contained all that was necessary to form new life. Semen, he thought, was strictly a catalyst for embryonic development and did not combine with the ovum in any way. Harvey, echoing Aristotle's notion of vital heat, compared the effect of sperm on egg as a "kind of contagion which the male communicates, almost as the lodestone does to iron." He added that "the woman, after contact with the spermatic fluid *in coitu,* seems to receive influence and to become fecundated without the cooperation of any sensible corporeal agent, in the same way as iron touched by the magnet is endowed with its powers and can attract other iron to itself." His conclusion did much to perpetuate the ancient myth of *aura seminalis,* that impregnation was due to an invisible vapor emanating from semen. Had Fabricius or Harvey examined semen with the magnifying lenses already at hand, they might have discovered spermatozoa, the tiny male sex cells with thin, motile tails. Seventy-seven years later, a medical student from the Netherlands made the momentous discovery, using nothing more complicated than a simple magnifying lens.

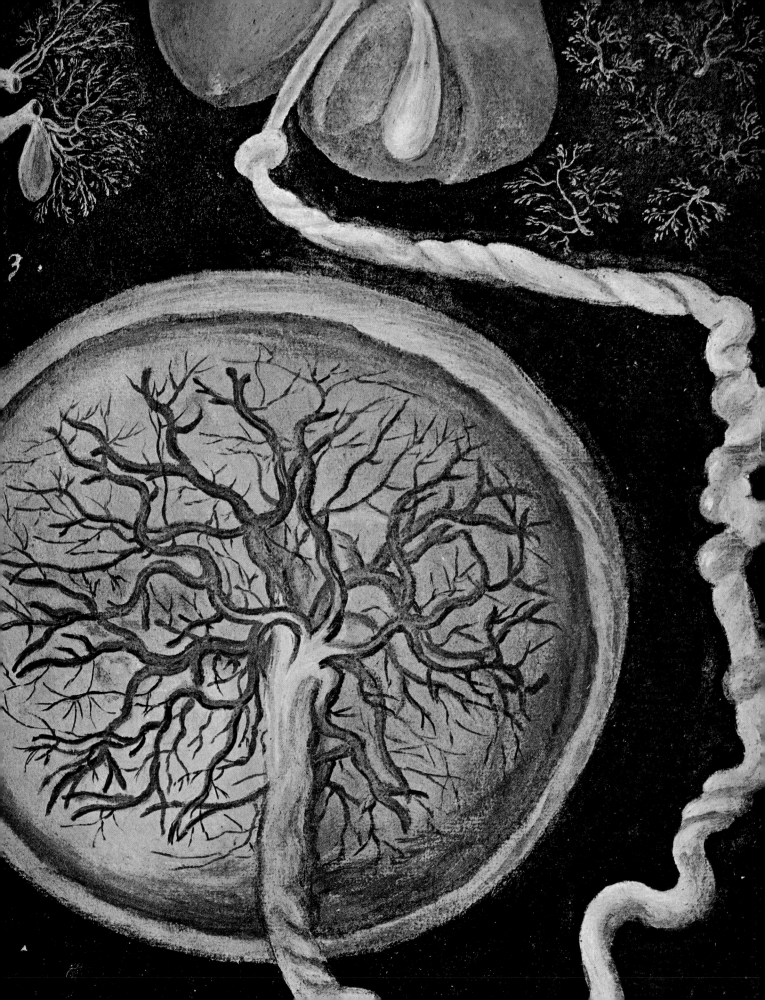

que la tête feroit peut-être plus grande à proportion du refte du corps, qu'on ne l'a deffinée icy.

Au refte, l'œuf n'eft à proprement appelle *placenta*, dont l'enfant, aprés y avoir demeuré un certain temps tout courbé & comme en peloton, brife en s'étendant & en s'allongeant le plus qu'il peut, les membranes qui le couvroient, & pofant fes pieds contre le *placenta*, qui refte attaché au fond de la matrice, fe pouffe ainfi avec la tête hors de fa prifon ; en quoi il eft aidé par la mere, qui agitée par la douleur qu'elle en fent, pouffe le fond de la matrice en bas, & donne par confequent d'autant plus d'occafion à cet enfant de fe pouffer dehors & de venir ainfi au monde.

L'experience nous apprend que beaucoup d'animaux fortent à peu prés de cette maniere des œufs qui les renferment.

L'on peut pouffer bien plus loin cette nouvelle penfée de la

Amid the hysteria that followed the discovery of the male sex cell in 1677, microscopists imagined seeing tiny men, animalcules, curled up inside each spermatazoon. This imaginative belief became medical dogma in the eighteenth century.

In 1677, Johan Ham van Arnhem, upon observing what he called "animalcules" in the semen of a patient suffering from venereal disease, brought the discovery to his mentor Anton van Leeuwenhoek, the greatest microscopist of his time. "These animalcules were smaller than the corpuscles which impart a red color to the blood," Leeuwenhoek observed, "so that I judge a million of them would not equal in size a large grain of sand. . . . I can best liken them in form to a small earthnut with a long tail. The animalcules moved forward with a snakelike motion of the tail, as eels do when swimming in water. . . . They lashed their tails some eight or ten times in advancing a hair's breadth."

Man the Animalcule

The discovery was made public the following year, prompting both awe and revulsion at so bewildering a concept. To some scientists, it seemed fantastic that so many sperm could take part in the formation of a single human being. But if only one of these creatures was responsible for fertilization, the pointless death of millions of others seemed contrary to any notion of a just divine plan. "I well know there are whole universities that won't believe there are living creatures in the male seed," Leeuwenhoek wrote, "but such things don't worry me, I know I'm in the right." Indeed, many of his colleagues believed that the sperm were only parasites, having arisen from putrefied matter. Those who did believe sperm were related to fertilization reported seeing a tiny man curled inside each spermatozoon. Others claimed to have seen minuscule horses galloping through the semen of a horse and long-eared animals in that of a donkey. Leeuwenhoek himself was not immune to the hysteria that followed the discovery. "Once I fancied I saw a certain form, about the size of a sand grain," he said, "which I could compare with some inward part of our body." In 1716, Leeuwenhoek wrote to a colleague, "Animalcules, too, differ in sex and are distinguished as male and female. Whence it would follow that if after marital copulation a male animalcule should reach that place in the [womb] provided for the reception of these animalcules, a male would be born, but if a female should have taken possession of that place a female would be born."

The belief that little men were curled up inside spermatozoa became medical dogma in the eighteenth century. Most people accepted as fact the time-worn assumption that the male sperm, the animalcule, was the seed and the female, the soil into which new life was planted. One hundred years after the discovery of spermatozoa, Italian biologist Lazzaro Spallanzani challenged the accuracy of seed and soil as metaphor for human reproduction. Questioning the proposition that animalcules were strange, tiny beings apparently living inside humans, he began unusual experiments to determine the role of the "spermatic worms." After fashioning a tiny pair of trousers from waxed fabric, he dressed male frogs and observed them trying to copulate with female frogs. The semen ejaculated during the unsuccessful attempts was caught inside the trousers. When the female frogs failed to conceive, he collected more semen and mixed it with the females' eggs in a small dish. It proved to be the first successful attempt at artificial fertilization. The fertilization of the frogs' eggs "was accomplished by means of the seminal liquor of the animals themselves," Spallanzani wrote, "and I have succeeded as well as if the male himself had performed his proper function." Spallanzani pressed on, experimenting with tree frogs to determine once and for all "whether the gross visible part of the seed be necessary to the fecundation of man and animals, or, whether the invisible attenuated part usually called the seminal vapor or aura, be destined to this purpose." He placed drops of seminal fluid from several toads on the bottom of a glass saucer. On the inside of the saucer's lid he attached twenty-six unfertilized frog's eggs directly above the fluid, but not touching it. He left the eggs in that position for five hours, allowing time for the semen to evaporate. The moisture that appeared on the eggs came from "the evaporated part of the seed." The eggs, he concluded, "had been bedewed with . . . the seminal aura." But the vapor did not fertilize the eggs, even in subsequent experiments, proving to Spallanzani, "that fecundation in the fetid toad is not the effect of the *aura seminalis*, but of the sensible part of the seed." Yet

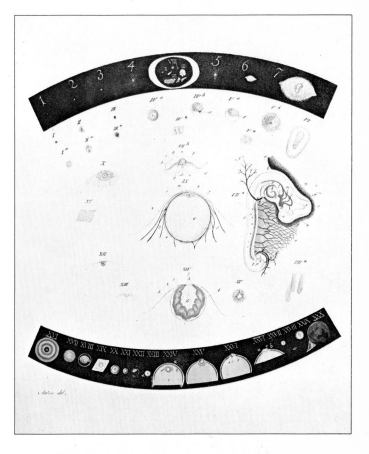

he obstinately refused to grant that sperm cells were a prime force in generation, attributing this to some other, unidentified element in seminal fluid. He believed this unknown element stimulated the growth of offspring, which must exist preformed in the egg. Spallanzani nevertheless brought the mystery of fertilization into science's bright light, and proved that eggs and semen, within the body or without, kindled life's spark.

In 1825, Swiss physician Jean-Louis Prévost theorized that spermatic animalcules were the essential element in the conception of new life and thought it "infinitely probable" that only one sperm was actually responsible for the formation of an embryo. It was not until 1827 that a thirty-five-year-old physician with a waning interest in bedside medicine found proof that mammals have internal eggs. Studying the ovaries of a dog through his microscope, Karl Ernst von Baer, professor of anatomical sciences at the University of Königsberg in Germany, discovered the ova quite by chance. "Led on more by inquisitiveness than by the hope of seeing the ovules," he wrote, "I was astounded when I saw an ovule . . . so plainly that a blind man could scarcely deny it. It is truly remarkable and astonishing that a thing so persistently and constantly sought and in all compendia of physiology considered as inextricable, could be put before the eyes with such facility." As enlightening as von Baer's discovery was, confusion persisted as to how semen acted upon an egg during fertilization. The intrusion of sperm into egg was difficult to observe, though many scientists tried. Finally, in 1843, English physician Martin Barry demonstrated the penetration of a rabbit's egg by sperm, though he erred in concluding how and precisely where fertilization took place.

After the middle of the nineteenth century, the cell, what German pathologist Rudolf Virchow deemed the "seat of life," became the center of scientific inquiry. Although it was commonly accepted that all cells arose from other cells, the precise mechanism of heredity was not understood. It was considered a phenomenon of growth in which offspring were fragmentations of both parents. Heredity was chiefly a concern of horticulturists and animal breeders, because economic necessity demanded better yields. For this reason, it was in orchards and on chicken farms that practical experiments were performed.

Heredity's Father

It was not until Gregor Mendel carried out his now famous experiments with the garden pea that the mystery of generation was replaced by scientific laws of heredity. Born in 1822 in Northern Moravia, Mendel entered the monastery at Brno, now in Czechoslovakia, at the age of twenty-one. Self-taught in mathematics and Greek, Mendel later studied the natural sciences at the University of Vienna. Upon his return to the cloister in 1853, he devoted more of his time to teaching and research. Mendel had always been fond of gardening. In his youth, he had experimented with cross pollinating flowers to produce new color varieties. The years of studying botany in Vienna had piqued Mendel's curiosity,

and so in the quiet monastery gardens he began his fateful research. He was keenly aware that what he pursued was nothing less than the secret of life. In 1854, five years before Charles Darwin published *Origin of Species*, Mendel had written: "It requires indeed some courage to undertake a labor of such far-reaching extent; this appears, however, to be the only right way by which we can finally reach the solution to a question the importance of which cannot be overestimated in connection with the history of the evolution of organic forms."

Mendel acquired a variety of pea strains from farms throughout Europe, growing thirty-four different varieties in the summer of 1854. The next year he examined the yield and chose seven characteristics for his experiments. Mendel found that smooth or wrinkled seeds produced plants with peas showing the same characteristics and that yellow or green seeds similarly grew plants with peas of like color. Crossing tall with short pea plants, he observed, resulted in roughly three tall plants and one short one. Crossing round and wrinkled seeds produced plants approximately three-quarters of which yielded round peas and one-quarter wrinkled ones. Beside the garden pea, Mendel conducted breeding experiments with pea weevils, mice and honeybees. He proposed the terms "dominant" and "recessive" to describe the characteristics that appeared more and less often, respectively. With adequately large numbers of plants, Mendel could actually predict the offspring's appearance with mathematical accuracy.

One cold February night in 1865, Mendel presented his results to forty scientists at the local society for natural sciences in Brno. His audience listened graciously to Mendel's hour-long talk on the hybridization of pea plants. Afterward the group of naturalists, astronomers, physicists and chemists applauded and left, without expressing the slightest inquisitiveness. Until the twentieth century, his work languished in obscurity.

In 1875, German embryologist Oskar Hertwig realized the significance for heredity of the union of nuclei in both sperm and egg, a phenomenon still not completely understood. Placing egg and sperm from sea urchins in a dish of sea water,

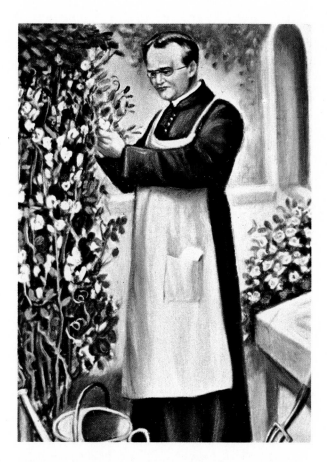

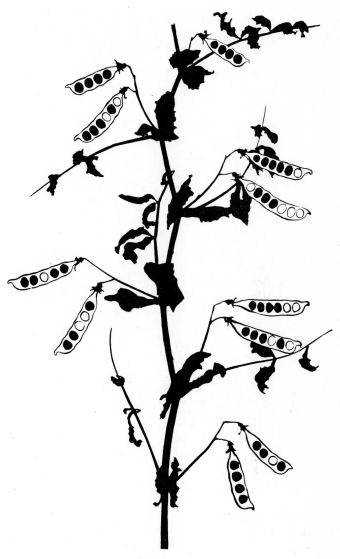

Hertwig watched a single sperm penetrate the ovum and observed the subsequent divisions of the chromosomes within the cells. Seventy-five years later in England, two scientists added a dimension to the understanding of heredity. Using the data from newly developed X-ray diffraction equipment, Francis Crick and James Watson at Cambridge University proposed the structure of deoxyribonucleic acid (DNA), the twisted double helix that is now known to contain all the information necessary to construct an entire living thing. Watson and Crick, bolstered by research conducted by earlier theorists, proved that during fertilization the combination of genetic material from the parents' sex cells establishes the unique characteristics of every human being.

The basis of all heredity is the gene, a small chain of nucleic acids responsible for constructing other molecules that power, maintain and govern the cell. Within each cell there are as

In the monastery gardens at Brno, now Czechoslovakia, Augustinian monk Gregor Mendel carried out his famous experiments in cross pollinating pea plants. By studying successive generations, Mendel deduced the laws of heredity upon which the modern study of genetics is based. With adequate numbers of plants, like the one shown in silhouette above, he could predict the offspring's characteristics with mathematical accuracy.

*The lion's mating sequence begins as
the male grimaces at the lioness,
which sometimes leads to a fight. If
she accepts his advances, the lioness
crouches in a copulation posture and
the pair mates.*

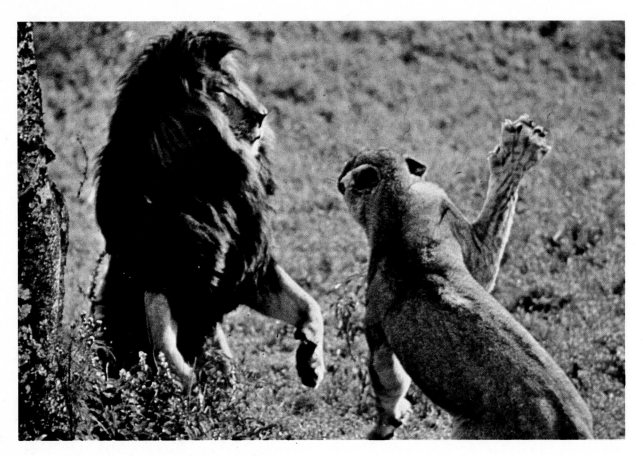

many as 100,000 genes grouped in chains called chromosomes. In combining during fertilization, these genes determine the hereditary characteristics that shape a new individual. As in Mendel's pea plants, dominant and recessive genes exist in the human genetic endowment. The gene coding for brown eyes is dominant over that for blue or gray eyes and the gene responsible for curly hair dominates the one for straight hair.

It is precisely this mixing of genes that makes possible an infinite variety of characteristics and talents necessary for survival in a changing environment. The combined genetic endowment of all the individuals in a species constitutes a constantly changing "gene pool." Sexual reproduction keeps the pool dynamic, according to genetic theory, and gives such organisms an evolutionary advantage over asexually reproducing creatures. This may be the reason sexual reproduction came about in the first place. Asexual reproduction, in which a parent duplicates itself exactly in its offspring, is an extremely conservative evolutionary trend. Faced with changes in the environment, static asexual forms are more prone to extinction than sexually reproducing organisms. Yet many simple forms of life still reproduce asexually. Bacteria simply divide in two, each offspring an identical but separate organism. Hydras, small freshwater polyps, can reproduce themselves from fragmented parts, budding new organisms that are exact replicas. Similarly, the pieces of a shattered flatworm can give rise to new, individual flatworms. While asexual reproduction is an efficient way to increase numbers, it limits diversity and flexibility.

The price of sexual reproduction is competition. Males and females seek mates, competing, sometimes ruthlessly, among themselves. In *The Descent of Man and Selection in Relation to Sex*, Charles Darwin reasoned that male peacocks are adorned with striking plumage to attract peahens. He believed that many characteristics of males of any species evolved as a means to "charm the females" or "to conquer other males in battle." Animal behaviorists think elaborate courtship rituals may serve a similar purpose. The female attempts to find the best father for her offspring by screening out the weak, unfit or philandering suitor. The doe, having captured the attention of a suitor, will turn tail and run over treacherous terrain in order to test his agility and swiftness. Periodically, she will stop and circle the buck, as if signaling approval, but when he attempts to mount her she runs off again. This ritual may allow the doe to assess her potential mate's strength, speed and endurance — all attributes that would make the buck a good mate and progenitor. Other animals, particularly some female birds, demand nests or gifts of food as proof of the male's devotion. In many species, courtship rituals consist of open and sometimes violent conflict among males. By the process of sexual selection, characteristics that prevail in the ritualistic competition for mates would tend to appear more often in subsequent generations. Among primates, sexual selection may explain why males are so often larger than females. Men are typically 20 to 30 percent heavier than women. The man's muscular limbs and larger skeletal framework are characteristics that would have made early human males particularly attractive as hunters and gatherers. It was to early woman's benefit to persuade such a man to provide food and animal skins and help care for offspring.

Judging the Gene

From the view of the new and controversial field of sociobiology, the gene is the basic unit of evolution and at the root of much individual and social behavior, including human. The riddle at the heart of sociobiology is that a particular form of social organization might give some members of a species an evolutionary advantage and thereby do the same work as a favorable gene. The influence of cultures, as well as genes, may ripple through the generations. Sociobiologists and their critics have locked horns in the eternal debate over nature and nurture.

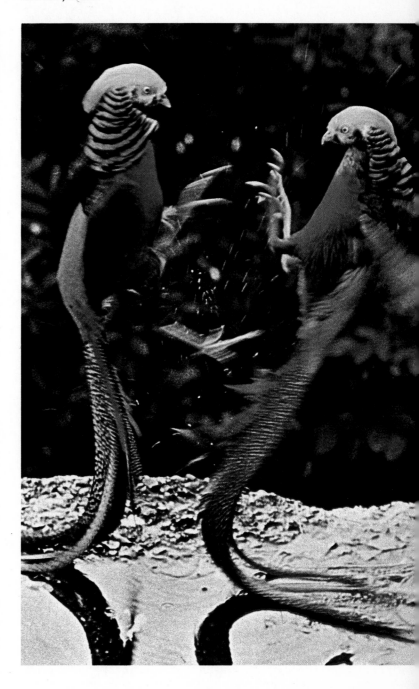

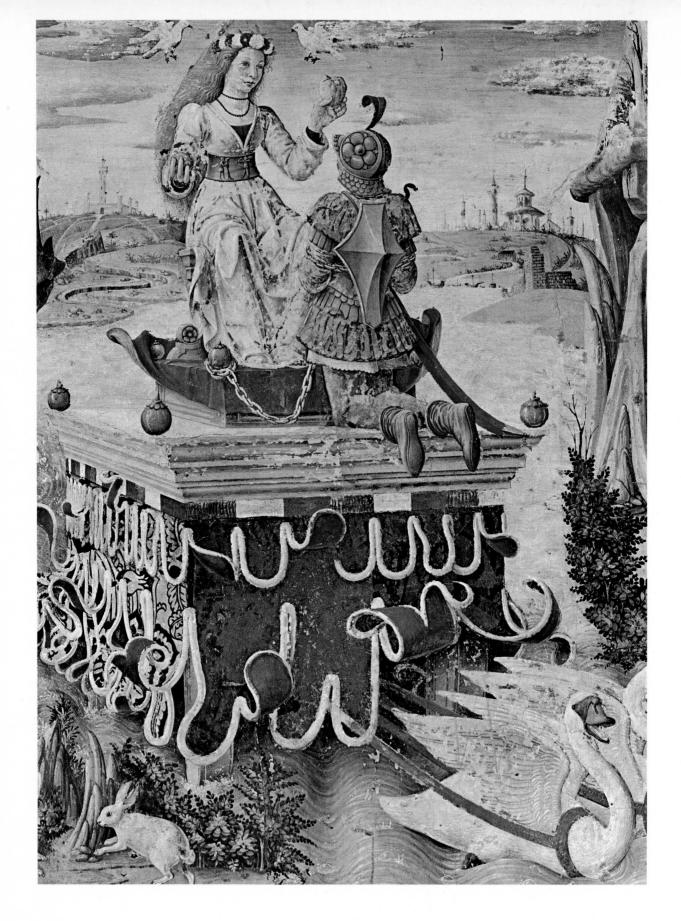

32

Sociobiologist Edward O. Wilson of Harvard
University sees genes at work in much human
behavior, including courtship and reproduction.
He theorizes that since a woman's egg is 85,000
times larger than a man's sperm cell, females
have a greater initial investment in sexual reproduction. In a lifetime, a woman can carry about
twenty ova through the cycle of fertilization,
gestation and birth. The cost of nurturing a fertilized egg within her body and caring for a baby
after birth far outweighs a man's biological investment. With each ejaculation, a man spends
200 to 500 million sperm, a tiny fraction of the
number he produces throughout his life. With
fertilization, his physical investment ceases.

Given this imbalance, in humans and other
species of animals, it pays for the female to be
coy, to protect her investment by being choosy
about whom she permits to fertilize her limited
supply of eggs. Some sociobiologists view the
human male's ritualistic gift giving, wooing and
entertaining in the same terms as courtship rituals found in other species of animals. The rites of
dating and engagement afford the human female
the same opportunity as the doe to measure her
prospective mate's potential as husband, father,
defender and provider. If particular traits are uni-
formly selected and progeny with those attributes flourish, then those genes will survive to be
passed on again. The characteristics consistently
not chosen will tend to disappear.

The loss of estrus, the period of ovulation or
heat, among human females, Wilson says, may
also have conferred an evolutionary advantage
by promoting pair bonding. Most animals can
only mate during the female's estrus, which in
many species occurs only once a year. During the
estrus, many female primates become sexually
aggressive. Their genitals swell and grow brightly
colored, and their bodies produce fatty acids that
lure and agitate the males. In troops of baboons,
males grow especially hostile when the females
of the troop are in heat.

The diffusion of estrus evenly throughout her
life, says Wilson, afforded the human female certain evolutionary benefits. More frequent sexual
activity between males and females cemented the
pair bond, says sociobiological theory, inducing

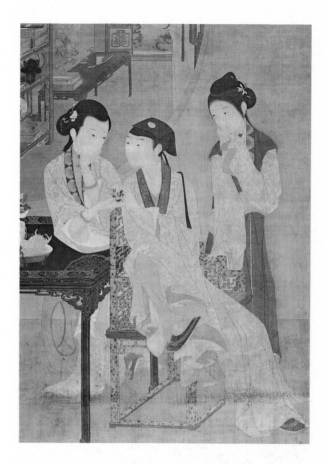

*Chinese lovers share a look that
spans all cultures in this eighteenth-
century painting of courtship.
The couple is joined by a maiden,
at right, who chaperoned for propriety's sake.*

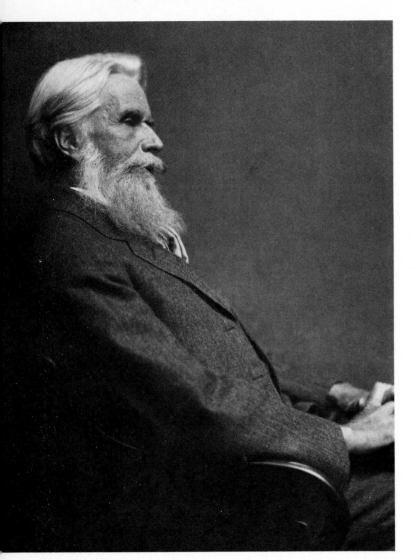

the male to stay with the female to provide for her and help raise offspring. Pair bonding also conferred evolutionary gains because two adults were better able than one to cope with the difficult physical environment, defend themselves against other animals and gather valuable resources. Whatever pleasure humans and other animals derive from sex, Wilson contends, is an evolutionary "means for inducing creatures with versatile nervous systems to make the heavy investment of time and energy required for courtship, sexual intercourse and parenting." Sociobiologists even suggest that the orgasm evolved as a positive reinforcement to motivate females into an active sex life and, so, cement the pair bond. "Human beings are unique among the primates in the intensity and variety of their sexual activity," according to Wilson. "Among other higher mammals they are exceeded in sexual athleticism only by lions." The king of beasts' prowess in such matters is remarkable. In Kenya, American field scientist George Schaller recorded a case in which one lion mated 157 times in two days, every twenty-one minutes on the average, without a morsel of food.

The Sexual Animal

A belief in the common heritage of animals and man is at the heart of both Darwin's theory of evolution and modern sociobiology. Darwin struggled with the dilemmas of nature and nurture, instinct and choice, as they appeared in many different forms of life. As the theories of Darwin and his successors reveal, no clear line separates biology from behavior, in all animals. At the end of the nineteenth century, just as science probed deeper into the mysteries of genetics and evolution, it also began to explore the sensitive subject of human sexuality.

While Victorian England still wrestled with the radical theories of Darwin, the ideas of another native son rocked English society. Psychologist Havelock Ellis studied not man's animal ancestors but what many people considered to be the animal still within. Sex was thought brutal and base. Ellis boldly declared "the person who feels that the sexual impulse is bad, or even low and vulgar, is an absurdity in the universe, an anoma-

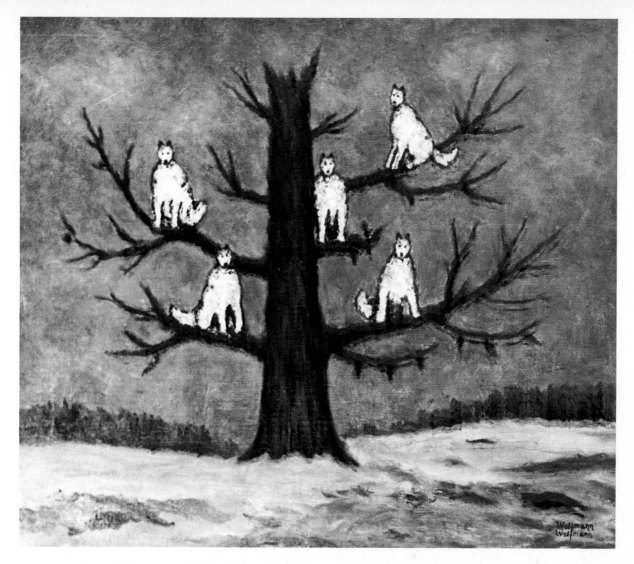

ly. He is like those persons in our insane asylums who feel that the instinct of nutrition is evil and so proceed to starve themselves." He advocated that should adults "privately consent to practice some perverted mode of sexual relationship, the law cannot be called to interfere." His *Studies in the Psychology of Sex,* published between 1897 and 1910, established the atmosphere for subsequent sexual theorizing. Tolerant of the sexually troubled and "inverted," Ellis himself had sexual problems. He was celibate until he was thirty-two years old and it was not until he was fifty-nine that he could respond sexually with anyone other than a stranger. By arguing that homosexuality was always inborn, Ellis tried to refute moral condemnation and statutes declaring such "inversions" illegal.

Ellis's theory of homosexuality opposed the ideas of the other great theorist of sexuality of the time, Austrian neurologist Sigmund Freud.

Perhaps Sigmund Freud's most famous case involved a patient known as the Wolf Man. While under Freud's care, he drew a picture of a particularly troublesome dream in which wolves terrorized him. Freud eventually concluded that a fear of castration beginning in early childhood held the key to understanding the patient's complex problem. In Freudian terms, the bare tree and menacing wolves are unmistakable allusions to the castration complex.

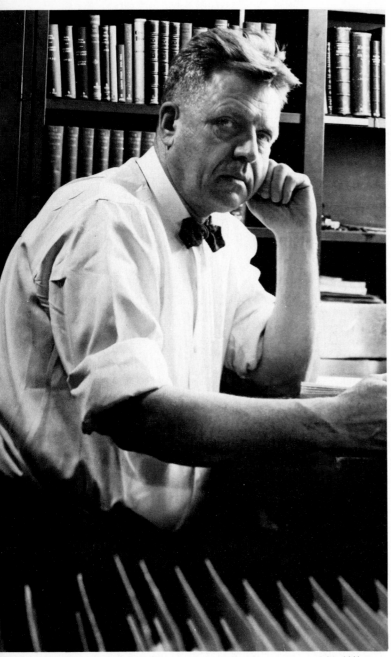

American sociologist and biologist Alfred Kinsey shocked the nation with his studies on human sexuality in the 1950s. His work revealed that Americans did not conform to many moral codes they professed.

Freud held that homosexuality was deeply rooted in the unconscious mind, a product of disturbing childhood episodes that later manifested themselves in a warped search for love.

Like Ellis, Freud could not tolerate the morality of his era because it "demands more sacrifices than it is worth." When he published *Three Essays on the Theory of Sexuality*, Freud did much to unveil what polite society had always kept secret. For Freud, symbols and dreams were paramount in analyzing the source of psychological disorders, which he believed had their origins in sexuality. Sexuality was the "indispensable premise" for mental illness. Through careful psychoanalysis, he believed, doctor and patient could discover the source of sexual problems.

Yet even in this age of science, myths about sexuality persisted. Freud believed that women experienced clitoral and vaginal orgasms. He held that sexual climax due to clitoral stimulation was immature, a relic of preadolescent discovery of sexual pleasure. In adulthood, he argued, women must transfer their sexual responsiveness from the infantile clitoris, or "masculine zone," to the vagina. In his view, women who failed to make the progressive step, though they may still have experienced orgasms, were "vaginally frigid." Freud's erroneous distinction pervaded sexual literature for seventy years.

Science and Sexuality

Unlike Freud, who argued that people dreaded and repressed the memories of their most significant sexual experiences, American sociologist and biologist Alfred Kinsey held a straightforward view of human sexuality. Kinsey was convinced that memory presented no meaningful hindrance to the examination of his patients' sexual histories. Between 1938 and 1953, Kinsey and his three associates amassed more than 16,000 individual sexual histories. Kinsey personally conducted almost half of the interviews. His promise of strict confidentiality, the reserving of moral judgments and his congenial approach during the interviews helped calm his subjects' initial qualms over recalling their most intimate sexual habits. What he learned exploded myths of sexuality long held true.

36

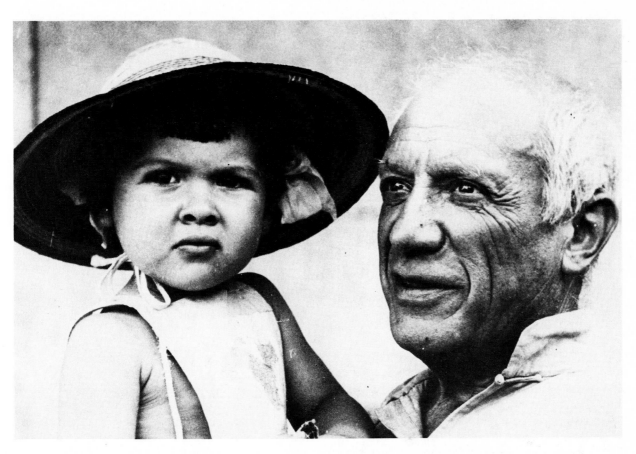

In *Sexual Behavior in the Human Male*, Kinsey revealed that most Americans masturbated. About half of the single population still masturbated at fifty years of age. Among women, many agreed that masturbation was "a desirable and often necessary" sexual outlet. He also found that about half of the married women and somewhat more men were sexually experienced before marriage. Still more remarkable, by forty years of age, 26 percent of the married women and half of the husbands said they had had an extramarital affair. There were "surprisingly few differences between the older and younger generations in these respects," Kinsey reported. Through interviews with thousands of subjects, he overthrew the popular notion that sexuality ceased during old age and challenged many other misconceptions about sexual preferences and behavior. It seemed the moral codes Americans had professed for years were not adhered to in practice.

Although the Kinsey studies were shocking for their time, the research of gynecologist William Masters and psychologist Virginia Johnson was more daring still. For the first time, a major university sponsored research in which hundreds of men and women, under controlled laboratory conditions, were monitored and their responses recorded during sexual intercourse. Masters led the study at Washington University in St. Louis in 1954. So concerned was he with establishing the respectability of his research that he enlisted the publisher of a major local newspaper and the commissioner of police as members of a special governing board to oversee the controversial experiments. Masters and Johnson interviewed more than 1,200 potential subjects for the study and selected 694 as participants.

The scientists compared the physiological responses of males and females to masturbation, intercourse and other kinds of sexual stimulation.

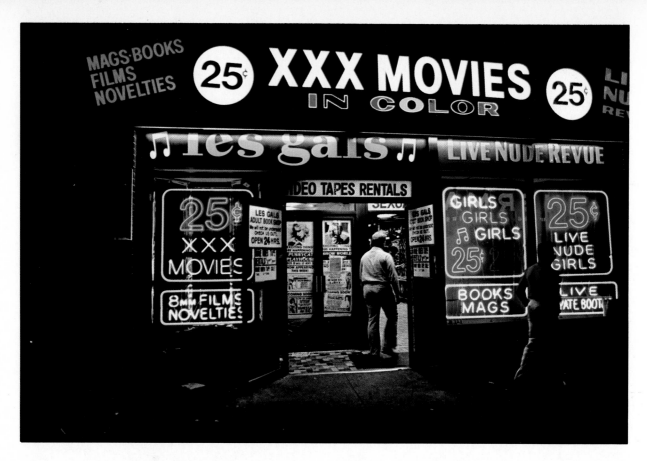

Their findings indicated that the human sexual response consisted of four phases: excitement, plateau, orgasm and recovery. Before their study and subsequent book, *Human Sexual Response*, almost nothing was known about the physiology of orgasm. They demonstrated that not only was female orgasm a physiological fact but that it was an experience involving the whole body. Masters and Johnson corrected Freud's theory of female sexual response. "From an *anatomic* point of view," they observed, "there is absolutely no difference in the response . . . to effective sexual stimulation, regardless of whether stimulation occurs as a result of clitoral area manipulation, natural or artificial coition, or for that matter, from breast stimulation alone."

They found that sexual cycles were not different for men and women, as had been held, but surprisingly similar. They concluded that Kinsey had erred in believing men were more excited by visual sexual stimulation than women. Masters and Johnson declared that masturbation was not harmful. As late as 1959, a survey of senior medical students at five Pennsylvania medical schools revealed that half thought masturbation led to insanity. Even more surprising, one in five of the professors believed it, too.

Prior to the work of Masters and Johnson, therapy for those with sexual problems meant long, drawn-out sessions with doctors and psychiatrists. As a result of their research, Masters and Johnson opened a clinic for sexual dysfunction. Their intensive two-week course of therapy often provided successful results. Masters has expressed his homage to Kinsey, the scientist who opened "the previously closed doors of our culture to definitive investigation of human sexual response." The comment could apply to his and Virginia Johnson's research as well, given its tremendous contribution to the understanding of both the physiological and psychological complexities of human sexuality. Before their studies, no medical school in the country offered courses in human sexuality. Now such courses are part of the standard curricula in many medical schools.

In the wake of Masters and Johnson's research, human sexuality became an important and respected field of medical and psychological inquiry. "It appears that sex research — like some kinds of sexual behavior — has come out of the closet," said psychiatrist Stanley F. Yolles in his opening address before the world's first workshop on future directions of sex research, held in 1974. "In the field of human sexuality," Yolles added, "we have the opportunity as well as a responsibility to shape the future."

The study of human sexuality today spans subjects like the supposed psychological differences between men and women and the influence of sexual mores in society. The brains of men and women, some scientists believe, are organized differently, allowing for specialized abilities between the genders. Eleanor Maccoby, chairman of Stanford University's psychology department, and Carol Jacklin, a Stanford research associate, suggest that in broad terms the brains of men seem organized in a way that emphasizes visual-spatial abilities, while women's brains generally afford them greater verbal skills. The theory has gained both supporters and detractors. The Stanford study has also mounted evidence to disprove myths that boys are more analytic than girls and that female infants respond differently than males to sound. Maccoby and Jacklin found no evidence supporting the notion that girls are more affected by heredity and boys, more by environment. "The two sexes learn with equal facility in a wide variety of situations," they concluded in *The Psychology of Sex Differences.* "If learning is the primary means by which the environment affects us, then the two sexes are equivalent in this regard."

The social issue at the heart of research into sexuality is the appropriateness or destructiveness of contemporary cultural mores. An exploration of morality and sexual attitudes is crucial for the formation of sound moral judgments, not only for lawmakers but for people in general. Contemporary sex research studies sexuality, sex roles, morality, the effects of pornography on society and many other explosive subjects. It strides into a corner of the human psyche where many fear to tread, and today engenders fascination and outrage no less than it did a century ago.

Still, modern science has only peeked beneath the veil that has obscured the fundamentals of sexuality and new life since earliest times. Today scientists can manipulate the seeds of life in genetic engineering laboratories around the world. But human conception and reproduction still partake of the mysterious spirit that the ancients saw in the sun, moon, earth and gentle rains.

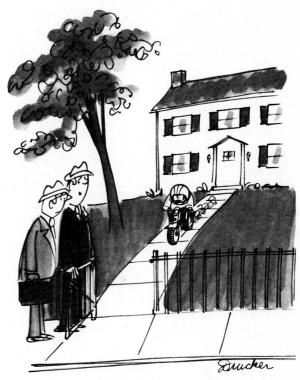

"My daughter Patience."

This cartoon parodies the controversy surrounding supposedly innate differences between females and males. The father's chagrin over his daughter's drag racing is both humorous and poignant.

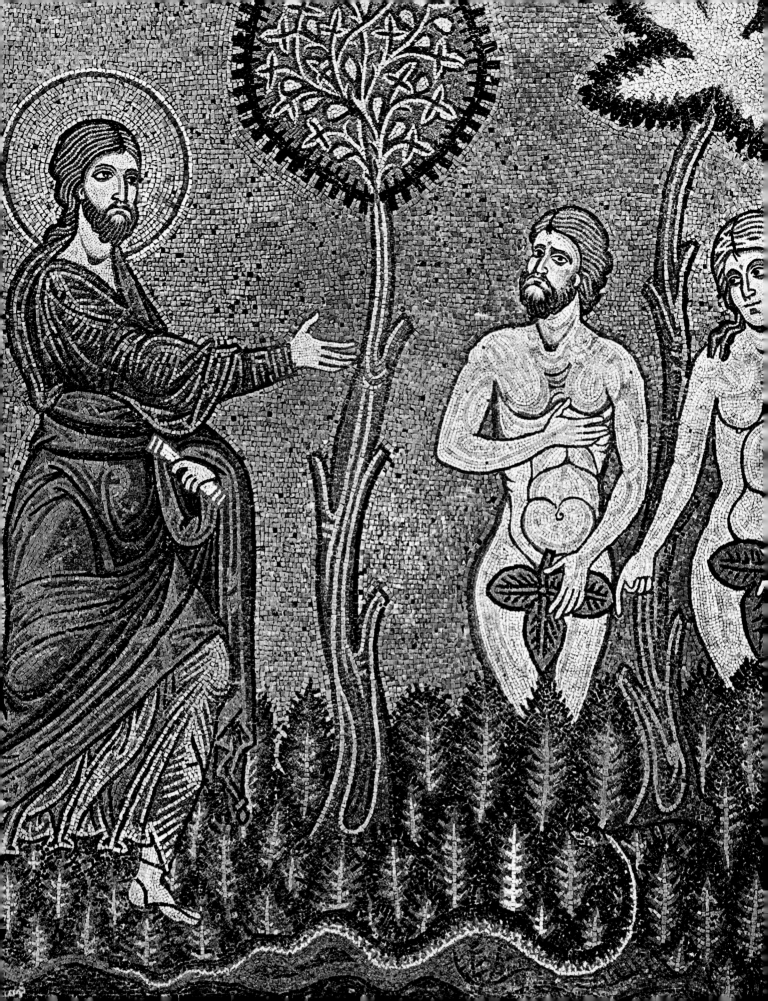

Chapter 2

The Seeds of Life

A nd they were naked, the man and his wife, and were not ashamed." So says the Book of Genesis, relating Adam and Eve's innocence in the fabled garden. After both tasted the forbidden fruit, "they knew that they were naked; and they sewed fig leaves together, and made themselves aprons."

Notwithstanding the biblical account, anthropologists doubt that man first wore clothes from a sense of shame. Even today, Eskimos disrobe completely inside their igloos. Japanese boatmen strip when it starts to rain, storing their clothes in a dry place. Caught in the fields without veils, Arab women may lift their skirts above their heads, thereby exposing what Westerners regard as a more private part of the anatomy.

Nor, apparently, are clothes designed for protection from the elements. Aboriginal Indians of Tierra del Fuego, the frigid tip of South America, wore only primitive shields, which they would occasionally shift to windward. Many anthropologists now believe that man began wearing clothes to protect his genitals from hostile magic, because he dwelled in a world heavily populated with spirits, good and bad. Whatever the reason, clothes are nearly universal. To the scientist, they hide organs of the most astonishing complexity.

Nature's grand plan for human reproduction relies on anatomical structures that dependably unite sperm and egg. At the lower rungs of the animal kingdom, among aquatic life, sperm is often conveyed in the pervasive medium of water. Some species, like salmon, build primitive nests for their fertilized eggs in the gravel of stream beds. Others, like the oyster, simply cloud the water with millions of eggs and sperm, hoping for the best. Male sharks have a pair of claspers protruding from their pelvic fins. These are inserted into a canal on the female that carries both waste and reproductive products. The vent is called the cloaca, Latin for "sewer."

Cast from paradise for tasting forbidden fruit, Adam and Eve are admonished by God in this mosaic from a thirteenth-century Italian church. Born of dust, man was condemned to "return unto the ground." Somewhere east of Eden, after the fateful expulsion, "Adam knew Eve his wife; and she conceived." So began, according to the Book of Genesis, the endless cycle of human generations.

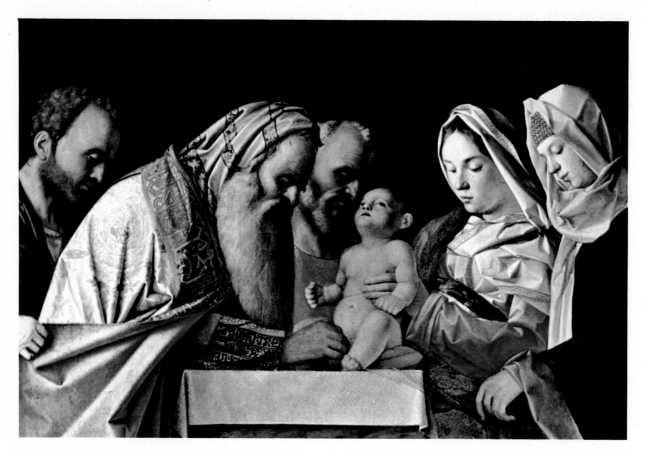

For land-dwelling creatures, a more sophisticated method is usually required. The mechanics of sperm transfer have led to the evolution of the penis. Some reptiles, including the crocodile, have organs that appear to be forerunners. But in mammals, the penis has reached its highest stage of refinement. The males of many species are fitted with a penile bone to make insertion easier. In dogs, the bone is rather simple in design, with a deep groove running its length for the urethra, a channel for sperm and urine. Among animals so equipped, the bones come in a variety of shapes. In the squirrel, the bone ends in a hemispheric plate that looks like a rooster's comb. The penile bone of a vole has clawlike prongs at its tip.

Every Man Child

Among mammals, only primates have penises that hang freely from the body wall. This feature confers a distinct evolutionary advantage, for many primates spend their lives hanging from branches. The penis's design enables muscles at its base to rid the body of urine efficiently. And of all primates, man alone does not have a penile bone. The adaptation prevents crippling fractures of the penis, because man's upright stature and bipedal gait expose the organ to danger.

At the tip of the penis lies the acorn-shaped glans, separated from the shaft by a rim of tissue called the corona, or crown. At birth, the glans is covered by the foreskin, a hood of tissue that can be retracted. In the United States, 80 percent of newborn boys are circumcised, a procedure that surgically removes the foreskin. Circumcision has a long history. The ritual was practiced in Egypt 6,000 years ago, possibly to mark slaves. Jews adopted the procedure, according to Genesis, when God told Abraham: "This is my covenant, which ye shall keep, between me and you and thy seed after thee; Every man child among you

The concerted energies of several glands and organs ensure that healthy sperm will encounter the female ovum. Columns of spongy tissue in the penis swell with blood during erection. Sperm are produced by the testicles, which hang in a pouch called the scrotum. Storage tanks, the epididymes consist of coiled tubes that the sperm navigate while they mature. Inside the long stem of the vas deferens, sperm are kept in suspended animation. Just before ejaculation, the seminal vesicles, prostate gland and Cowper's gland all contribute substances that nourish sperm and lower the acidity of the vagina.

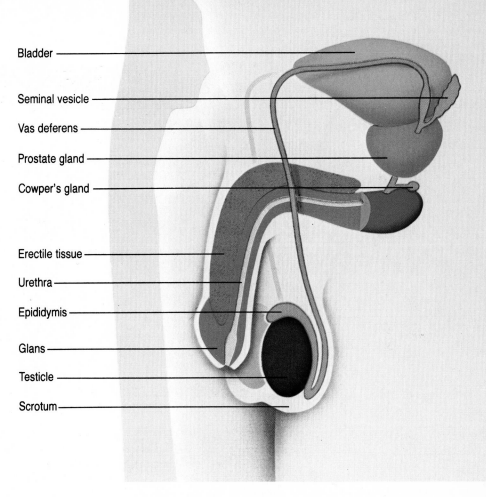

Bladder

Seminal vesicle

Vas deferens

Prostate gland

Cowper's gland

Erectile tissue

Urethra

Epididymis

Glans

Testicle

Scrotum

shall be circumcised." For centuries, in Western countries, Jews kept the covenant while Gentiles went uncircumcised. In the Victorian era, an age marked by sexual repression and intolerance, circumcision was thought to prevent masturbation, which was widely believed to cause insanity. In 1893, one British doctor claimed that the foreskin caused hysteria, epilepsy, "nocturnal incontinence" and irritation that might "give rise to erotic stimulation." Advocating the practice, another doctor attributed longer life, better health, calmness and fewer doctor bills to circumcision.

Since that time, doctors have learned that the mental health argument is groundless. At least in the United States, circumcision remains the rule because it probably prevents penile cancer and simplifies hygiene by making the glans easier to clean. Nevertheless, penile cancer is an exceedingly rare disease. Outside the United States, the operation is becoming increasingly rare, except

where cultural or religious tradition requires it — in Israel, Arab countries and among some tribes in sub-Saharan Africa. The American Academy of Pediatrics has recently concluded, "There is no absolute medical indication for routine circumcision of the newborn."

Hanging below the penis is the scrotum, a pouch that contains the testicles, two egg-shaped organs that manufacture sperm. In 75 percent of men, the left testicle hangs slightly lower than the right. Some scientists think the uneven positioning may prevent the testicles from jostling each other during ordinary movement. Because normal body temperature is too warm for the production of sperm, the testicles must be suspended. Temperature in the testicles averages about 3° to 5° F below body temperature. A muscular response in the scrotum operates like a thermostat, keeping the temperature constant. In cold weather, the scrotum contracts and the testi-

Minute factory lines, thousands of seminiferous tubules in the testicles manufacture sperm. Sertoli cells nourish embryonic germ cells, which divide and become full-fledged sperm as they progress toward the tube's center. Like quality control inspectors, the watchful Sertoli cells also weed out defective sperm. Despite such errors, the sperm industry is remarkably prolific — every day up to 500 million are made.

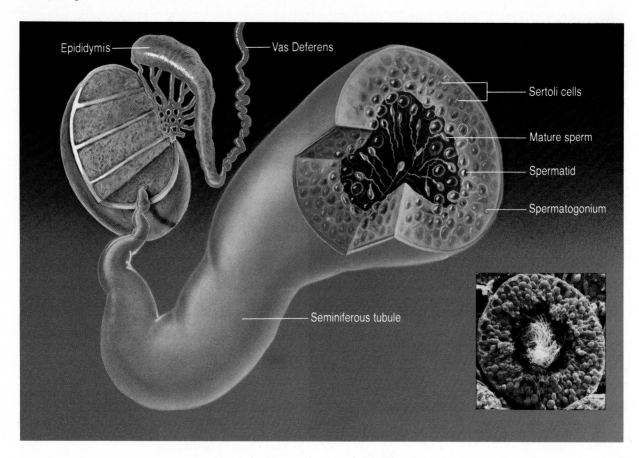

Epididymis — Vas Deferens

Sertoli cells

Mature sperm

Spermatid

Spermatogonium

Seminiferous tubule

cles are drawn toward the body, where they are warmed. Researchers have implanted the testicles of animals in their abdomens, thereby raising the testicular temperature a few degrees, enough to stop sperm production. Returned to the scrotum, the testicles resume the production of sperm.

Packed into each testicle are about one thousand seminiferous tubules, factory lines where sperm production occurs. When unraveled, each tube is about thirty inches long. Lining the tubes are spermatogonia, parent cells for sperm which puberty stirs into action. Over a lifetime, a man produces an astounding number of sperm, perhaps as many as twelve trillion. All sperm are descended from only one or two thousand spermatogonia that migrate into the embryonic testicles during pregnancy. In the first step of sperm production, a spermatogonium divides. One cell stays behind for future divisions. The other moves into a layer of specialized cells in the tube.

Called Sertoli cells after the nineteenth-century Italian physiologist who first described them, these cells nurse the germinal sperm cell by providing nutrients. Sertoli cells also secrete fluid that fills the tubes, creating an outward flow. At this stage, the germinal cell, like all other human cells, still has forty-six chromosomes carrying the coded information needed to create life. After another division, the cell doubles its chromosomes. Dividing twice more, the cell has become four spermatids, in the process called meiosis. Spermatids harbor twenty-three chromosomes, one-half the human code. Each carries an X chromosome, which will make a girl at fertilization, or a Y chromosome, which will make a boy.

Under further tending from Sertoli cells, each spermatid is transformed into a full-fledged spermatozoon. The nucleus becomes compact and oval-shaped. What remains of the spermatid develops into a neck and long tail. From the seminiferous tubules, the newborn sperm move into the epididymis, one lying atop each testicle. The epididymis is a storage tank, each of which contains about twenty feet of coiled tube. Like ships passing through a canal, the sperm navigate the epididymis in about ten days as they mature. Once they complete the passage, the sperm then climb the vas deferens, a long tube connecting each testicle to a seminal vesicle behind the bladder. Sperm negotiating the vas deferens release carbon dioxide, creating a mildly acidic environment that keeps them in a state of suspended animation. In all, it takes about seventy-four days for a spermatogonium to become a mature spermatozoon. In the epididymes and vasa deferentia, they remain fertile for several weeks. If not ejaculated, they eventually degenerate and are absorbed by the body.

The Testosterone Industry

The manufacture of sperm is sparked and regulated by hormones. Together, these chemical messengers govern many functions, including growth, salt balance and digestion. The hormones epinephrine and norepinephrine are secreted by glands near the kidney in response to fear, pain and muscle exertion. They divert blood to the muscles and boost the level of blood sugar. When blood sugar reaches too high a level, the pancreas releases the hormone insulin, which enables cells to absorb the excess. Diabetics suffer from an inability to manufacture sufficient insulin or to release it properly from the pancreas.

At puberty, the testicles secrete testosterone, a hormone that triggers various physiological changes in the male. As the testosterone level rises, the larynx becomes longer, deepening the voice. Gradually the shoulders become broader and beard growth is stimulated. In tandem with growth hormone, testosterone also promotes the body's growth. Around the age of twenty, the hormone stops the growth of long bones. It is an exquisite bit of timing. When growth ceases, men reach their sexual peak, avoiding competition between the two processes.

Some research has suggested a definite link between testosterone and aggression. In the late 1970s, Rutgers University psychologist June

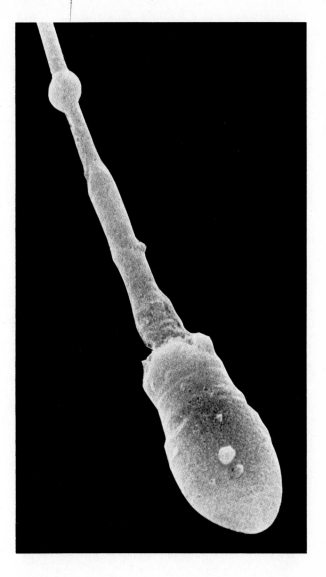

45

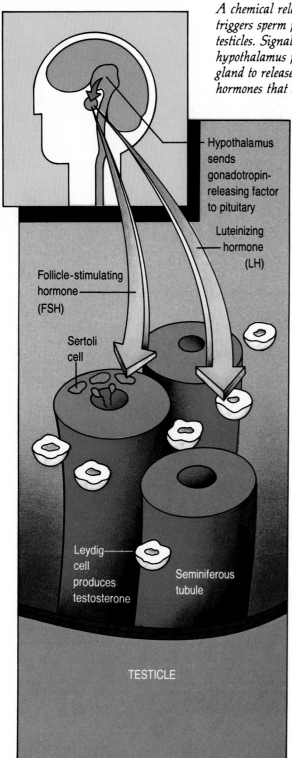

A chemical relay of hormones triggers sperm production by the testicles. Signals from the brain's hypothalamus prod the pituitary gland to release FSH and LH — hormones that travel through the blood to the testicles. LH commands cells to make testosterone, another hormone, below in crystal form. Testosterone develops male features like body hair and, in concert with FSH, coordinates sperm production.

Hypothalamus sends gonadotropin-releasing factor to pituitary

Luteinizing hormone (LH)

Follicle-stimulating hormone (FSH)

Sertoli cell

Leydig cell produces testosterone

Seminiferous tubule

TESTICLE

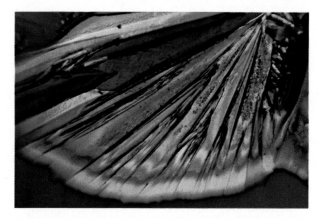

Reinisch studied the children of women who, in the 1960s, had taken a drug having testosterone-like effects. The drug had been administered during pregnancy to prevent miscarriage. Reinisch described six provocative situations to the children, such as being pushed out of place in a line. When asked what they would do, overwhelmingly, these children responded more aggressively than their brothers and sisters. Reinisch believes that testosterone somehow adds "flavor," increasing individualism, self-assurance and "perhaps even the propensity for violent behavior." Many scientists, however, remain highly skeptical of Reinisch's findings. In particular, they point to the girls born of the mothers who took the drug. These girls had enlarged clitorises that looked like small penises. In the ensuing confusion, their parents raised them as tomboys. Many scientists insist that such cultural factors explain the heightened aggressive behavior.

Despite this controversy, scientists generally agree that testosterone is fundamentally linked to violence. As evidence, they argue that violent, senseless crimes are almost never committed by women. Moreover, violent criminals treated with drugs that lower testosterone levels sometimes lose their aggressive tendencies. One doctor cites the case of a nineteen-year-old man who was shot while fleeing a bank he had just robbed. The wound cost the man both testicles. Afterward, he became less violent. A model prisoner, he was paroled within a few years. After he married, he consulted the doctor because his sex drive was waning. In all other respects, he appeared happily married and well adjusted. Although a testicle transplant proved impractical, the man was treated with synthetic testosterone. Six months later, he was in prison for robbing another bank.

Testosterone production is coordinated by a remarkable relay of chemical commands that begin with the stimulation of nerve cells in the brain. Once stirred, these neurons release small neurotransmitter molecules that migrate to the hypothalamus, a structure at the core of the brain. On cue, the hypothalamic cells secrete their supply of a hormone called gonadotropin-releasing factor. The hormone flows along a system of small veins and capillaries to the pituitary gland, a tireless center of hormone production, just a few centimeters away. Scientists learned about the ties between the hypothalamus and the pituitary gland when they implanted small electrodes in the brains of experimental animals. By burning minute lesions into the hypothalamus, the researchers found that the pituitary stopped secreting hormones. Likewise, they also discovered that electrical stimulation of hypothalamic cells dramatically raised hormone levels.

At the pituitary gland, gonadotropin-releasing factor causes the pituitary to release two more hormones, luteinizing hormone (LH) and follicle-stimulating hormone (FSH). These chemical messengers then enter the blood stream and are carried to the testicles. LH binds to receptor sites on Leydig cells, which lie in nests between the sperm-producing tubes of the testicles. Receptor sites are target molecules on cells that precisely fit specific chemicals like pieces of a jigsaw puzzle. This coupling initiates chemical reactions that eventually command the cells' machinery to make testosterone. In the same way, FSH binds to receptors on the Sertoli cells, regulating sperm production in concert with testosterone.

Most testosterone released into the blood is chemically bound to a plasma protein. These molecules render the hormone inert. Unbound testosterone molecules survive up to thirty minutes, after which they are converted to various derivative chemicals. Scientists believe protein-bound testosterone provides a strategic reserve of the hormone, ready for deployment when the testosterone level fluctuates. Fortunately, the system seldom goes awry. The testosterone industry is regulated by an ingenious feedback mechanism that keeps hormone levels steady. After LH triggers testosterone production, the testosterone chemically suppresses the secretion of releasing factor by the hypothalamus. This action dampens the release of LH by the pituitary. If testosterone levels run high, LH production temporarily shuts down. When the testosterone level begins to fall, releasing factor and LH trigger increased production. A similar cycle regulates the manufacture of FSH, but scientists have not identified the precise mechanism. The testicles make a substance that scientists have labeled inhibin, which may suppress FSH secretion.

When a man's testicles are removed before puberty, the scheduled release of testosterone never occurs. Body hair and whiskers never sprout, the penis remains boyish and the voice keeps a high pitch. Castration after puberty does not reverse all physical changes of adolescence. Although erection is still possible, interest in sex dwindles.

Throughout history, castrated men, eunuchs, have been prized as guardians of royal harems. Greek general and writer Xenophon recorded that the Persian monarch Cyrus the Great "selected eunuchs for every post of personal service to him, from the doorkeepers up." Praising the policy, he added that "no one has ever performed acts of greater fidelity in his master's misfortunes than eunuchs do."

In China, thousands of eunuchs tended the emperors of the Ming Dynasty, founded in 1368 and lasting nearly three centuries. When China's last emperor, Pu Yi, was deposed in 1924, the imperial complement of eunuchs numbered only two hundred. Despised by the Chinese as "court rats" who arbitrarily wielded power, the eunuchs were taunted on the streets and forced to beg for money. Today, no more than three survive, sad relics of an almost forgotten era. Eighty-year-old

Sun Yaoting was castrated by his father in 1912 and learned the palace rituals of kowtowing, or bowing, to superiors and filling the emperor's water pipe. Reflecting on his youth he recalls, "My happiest day was when I was transferred to the empress's chamber. Now I have nothing left. Not even her picture."

Juvenal, first-century poet and satirist, recorded the vices of the Roman Empire, noting that eunuchs were avidly sought by Roman women as lovers, partly because there was "no worry about abortions." Flavian Emperor Domitian eventually prohibited castration. In time, centuries later, eunuchs were more admired for their soprano voices than their amatory talents. The papal choir of the Sistine Chapel was filled with eunuchs until 1878, when Pope Leo XIII ended the tradition.

A Woman's Body

Although Henry Higgins, the exasperated professor in *My Fair Lady,* once cried "Why can't a woman be more like a man?" such an arrangement would not profit our species. Evolution demands two sexes, the better to stir the genetic pot through reproduction. Nowhere are the differences between men and women more pronounced than in reproductive anatomy.

Of necessity, the female reproductive system is differently designed from the male's. The male role ends with the production of sperm and their delivery to the female. Women must produce eggs, shelter and nourish the developing fetus, and successfully deliver a child. Corresponding to the male testicles are ovaries, two almond-shaped organs about one-and-a-half inches long that lie midway between the vagina and navel. The ovaries produce female hormones, which trigger physiological changes, like breast growth, at puberty. They also ripen the ovaries' ova, the eggs, which become fertilized when penetrated by sperm. Leading from the ovaries are two thin ducts called Fallopian tubes, which meet at the pear-shaped uterus, or womb. During pregnancy, the womb shelters the fetus and enlarges to accommodate its growth. The outer wall is thick with muscle tissue that will expel a baby at birth. The narrow end of the uterus, pointing downward, is the cervix, a thick muscular opening.

A woman's external sex organs are no less complex. Enclosing the genitals are two folds of tissue resembling lips, the labia majora. Lying above them is a mound of fatty tissue, the mons pubis, which cushions the man's and woman's pubic bones during intercourse. Beneath the labia is another pair of lips, the labia minora. Unlike the outside pair, they are not covered with pubic hair. In some women, they are larger than the labia majora, and may protrude slightly. In all women, the labia minora house oil and sweat glands. At the apex of the inner lips, buried in muscle and fibrous tissue, is a small bud of tissue called the clitoris. Descended from the same embryonic structure that becomes the male penis, the clitoris is among the most sensitive organs in a woman's body. Like the penis, it swells with blood during sexual arousal. Only in a few women, however, does it become fully erect. In many animal species, females have the equivalent of a penile bone. Cats, seals and rodents, among others, have both penile and clitoral bones.

In some Moslem countries, including Egypt and the Sudan, the clitoris is surgically removed and the labia minora sewn together between the ages of eight and ten. The custom has a long tradition. The Greek geographer Strabo noted in the first century B.C. that, in addition to circumcising men, Egyptians "excised" women. The purpose of excision seems, at least partly, to assure sexual passivity and discourage promiscuity in women. According to a recent survey by a family planning agency in Cairo, 90 percent of the women interviewed had had part of the clitoris and labia minora removed. When the woman marries, the small opening left to allow menstrual bleeding is slightly widened to permit intercourse.

Encircled by the labia, the vagina doubles as port of entry for the penis and exit for the baby. A muscular tube four to six inches long, the vagina is normally collapsed. During intercourse, its walls adapt to the penis. At its outer gate is a thin membrane called the hymen. Although traditionally considered the badge of virginity, the hymen often ruptures in childhood through normal play and activity. Usually the tissue is broken in a woman's first intercourse. If thin, it may break painlessly. Sometimes, however, the hymen is so

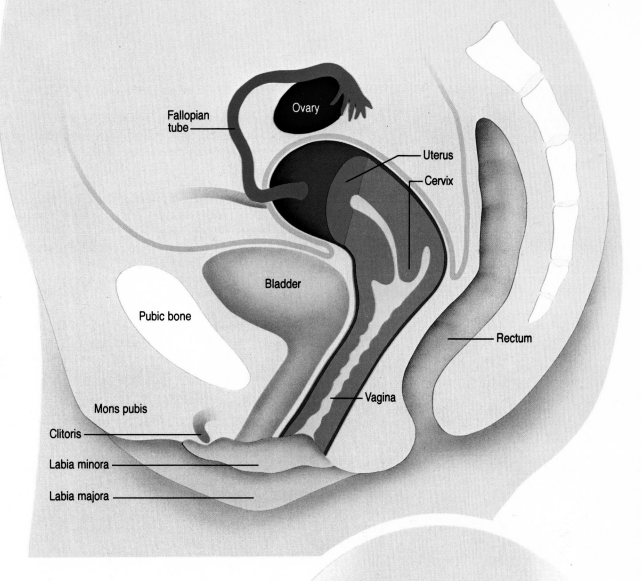

Fallopian tube

Ovary

Uterus

Cervix

Bladder

Pubic bone

Rectum

Mons pubis

Vagina

Clitoris

Labia minora

Labia majora

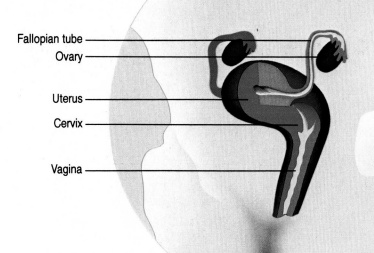

Fallopian tube

Ovary

Uterus

Cervix

Vagina

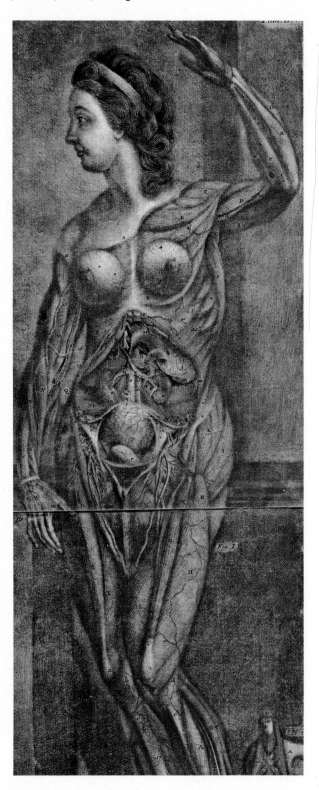

tough that it must be cut surgically. Nevertheless, women occasionally reach the delivery room with their hymen still intact.

Virginity has long been prized. In the Sumerian *Epic of Gilgamesh,* the citizens of Uruk resented their king's demand that he "be first with the bride." In what is now Cambodia, fourteenth-century Buddhist monks would customarily deflower virgins about to be married. In Islam, believers are said to be rewarded with 10,000 virgins when they reach paradise. Deflowered each night, the virgins will awaken every morning with their hymens miraculously restored. Eighty percent of Japanese men still insist on marrying virgins. Every year, about 35,000 operations are performed in Japan to restore broken hymens. Because the artificial substitute dissolves within a month, a delay in the wedding date means the surgical procedure must be repeated.

Seasons and Their Cycles

But more crucial to reproduction than a woman's virginity is the monthly readying of an ovum. In the female fetus, about 2,000 amoebalike germ cells, or oogonia, migrate toward the ovaries of the embryo from the yolk sac. These cells multiply. At birth, the baby's ovaries contain nearly 600,000 cells called oocytes, all descended from the oogonia. Oocytes reside in small sacs known as primordial follicles. Each oocyte has the potential, when fertilized, to develop into a child, but only about 400 will ever ripen. Most degenerate through adolescence and into adulthood.

The awakening of a woman's reproductive powers begins around the age of eight. For reasons not fully undersood, the hypothalamus begins secreting gonadotropin-releasing factor. The molecules migrate on a short path of capillaries to the pituitary gland and stimulate the secretion of the hormones FSH and LH. Released into the blood stream, they journey to the ovaries and kindle the production of the female hormone estrogen, testosterone's chemical cousin.

Gradually, the potent hormone incites physiological changes in the body. External genitalia — clitoris, mons pubis, labia and vagina — grow. The pelvis broadens to accommodate future demands of pregnancy and childbearing. Maturing

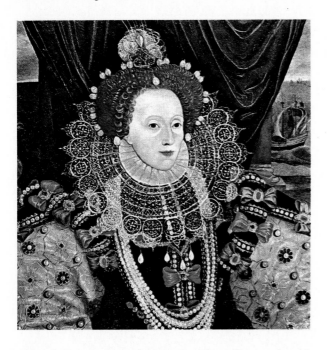

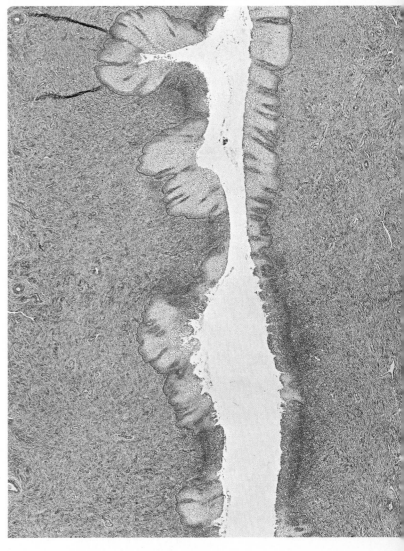

Fallopian tubes proliferate with cells equipped with waving cilia, miniature oars that create a current of fluids moving toward the uterus. In the years following the onset of puberty, the uterus itself increases two or three times in size. Like testosterone, estrogen spurs growth by boosting the activity of osteoblasts — cells that form bone. Later, the hormone causes the closing of the ends of the body's long bones. Just as in the male, competition between growth and reproduction is avoided. This phenomenon is more powerful in women than men. Female growth ceases several years before men stop growing.

During this metamorphosis, estrogen also prompts deposits of fat in the breasts, buttocks and thighs. Scientists now believe that fat plays a major role in triggering the monthly ovarian cycle. At the initial stages of adolescence, a woman's body has a five to one ratio of lean to fat tissue. At menarche, the first menstrual period, the ratio is three to one — a leap of 125 percent in just two or three years. Over the next one or two years, menstruation is irregular. Ovulation, the ripening of ova, does not occur. By the time monthly ovulation becomes firmly established, 28 percent of the body is fat tissue. Pregnancy consumes 50,000 calories, and milk production,

Normally collapsed, the vagina is flexible, adapting to the penis during intercourse. Sex researchers Masters and Johnson have learned that beads of lubricant appear on the vagina's walls in sexual arousal.

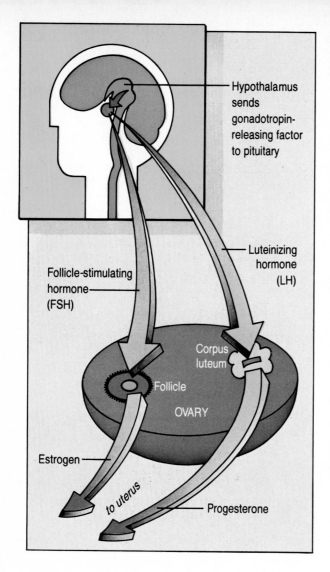

Hypothalamus sends gonadotropin-releasing factor to pituitary

Luteinizing hormone (LH)

Follicle-stimulating hormone (FSH)

Corpus luteum

Follicle

OVARY

Estrogen

to uterus

Progesterone

Stirred by FSH from the pituitary gland, ovaries develop ova, which lie in follicles. FSH also commands the follicles to make estrogen, a hormone that quickens the pituitary's release of LH. About two weeks into the ovarian cycle, a surge of LH bursts the follicle, releasing the ovum into a Fallopian tube. A blood clot forms on the abandoned follicle, which soon becomes a corpus luteum, a new structure that will churn out the hormone progesterone.

Fallopian tube

1,000 calories per day. Because 28 percent fat composition in a woman of average size equals about 99,000 calories, fat stores are sufficient to nourish a fetus through pregnancy and to nurse the baby for a month. Scientists speculate that a critical weight and fat composition, like a trip wire, start monthly ovulation.

The ovarian cycle starts with a wave of FSH secretion from the pituitary. The ovaries respond to the chemical signal. About fifteen or twenty follicles, each harboring an oocyte, awaken from their slumber of many years. The growing follicles, prodded by FSH, begin secreting estrogen. In a negative feedback loop, estrogen dampens the release of additional FSH. In a poorly understood manner, estrogen slows and then quickens LH secretion. The LH then commands the follicle to secrete more estrogen. The tempo of the follicle's growth quickens. A crust of granular cells thickens and bathes each oocyte in fluid.

Just before ovulation, each oocyte divides. Chromosomes are equally shared between the two new cells. But one cell snares most of the cytoplasm of the original cell and becomes a secondary oocyte. The other daughter cell clings to the new oocyte to become a polar body. This peculiar division with its unequal sharing of resources has a special purpose. After its release from the ovary, the secondary oocyte, now a mature ovum, drifts down toward the uterus at a leisurely pace, taking as long as ten days. By claiming the bulk of the nutrients, the ovum packs enough food to temporarily nourish an embryo if fertilization occurs.

One follicle outpaces its sisters. Thirteen days into the menstrual cycle, a surge of LH causes the mature follicle, now lodged against the ovary's wall, to swell. Badly weakened from enzymes secreted by the swelling follicle, the wall bursts on the fourteenth day. Some women actually feel a

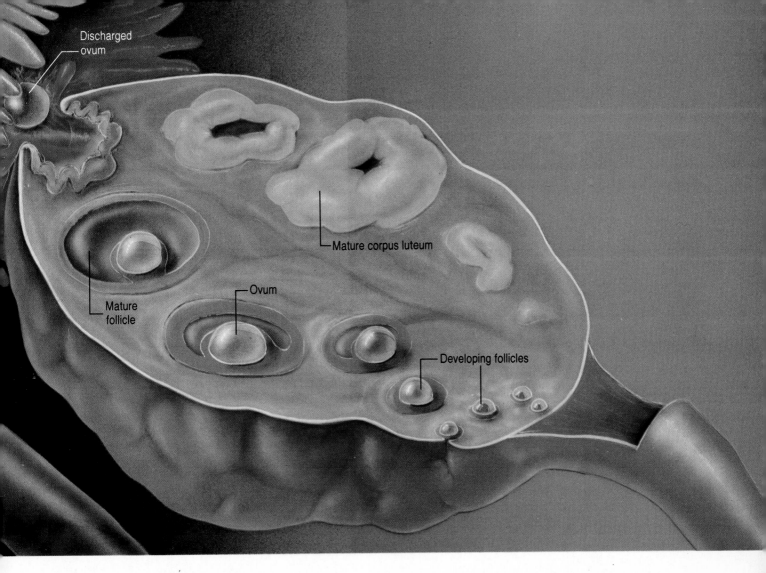

Discharged ovum

Mature corpus luteum

Ovum

Mature follicle

Developing follicles

twinge of pain, called *mittelschmerz,* as this happens. A rush of escaping fluid launches the ovum into the waiting arms of the Fallopian tube, which has enveloped the section of the ovary where the follicle has been growing. Beating cilia that line the tube create a current, sucking the ovum along on its passage to the womb.

The nineteen or so sister follicles that never fully developed shrink inside the ovary and die. Abandoned by the ovum, the follicle fills with blood. A clot forms, soon to be absorbed by follicle cells, which undergo rapid physical and chemical changes. The follicle becomes a new structure called the corpus luteum, Latin for "yellow body." A hormone factory, the corpus luteum shoulders the burden of estrogen production, and secretes two new hormones — relaxin and progesterone. Relaxin inhibits uterine contractions during pregnancy, preventing the onset of labor before full term. The other hormone,

progesterone, stimulates breast enlargement by fostering the development of milk sacs in anticipation of pregnancy. Through negative feedback, progesterone also checks further manufacture of FSH and LH. This event is neatly timed. If FSH and LH were released at this juncture in the ovarian cycle, they would stimulate new follicle maturation in the ovary. Because the corpus luteum secretes progesterone, ovulation will temporarily cease during pregnancy.

Meanwhile, hormones have quietly been preparing the womb for implantation of a fertilized egg. Early in the ovarian cycle, secretions of estrogen stimulate the endometrium, the innermost lining of the uterus. The lining gradually grows thick with cells, glands and blood vessels. After ovulation, fresh surges of progesterone from the corpus luteum stir endometrial cells, which swell and become corpulent. Glands on the lining twist into convoluted tubes and secrete a rich mucus.

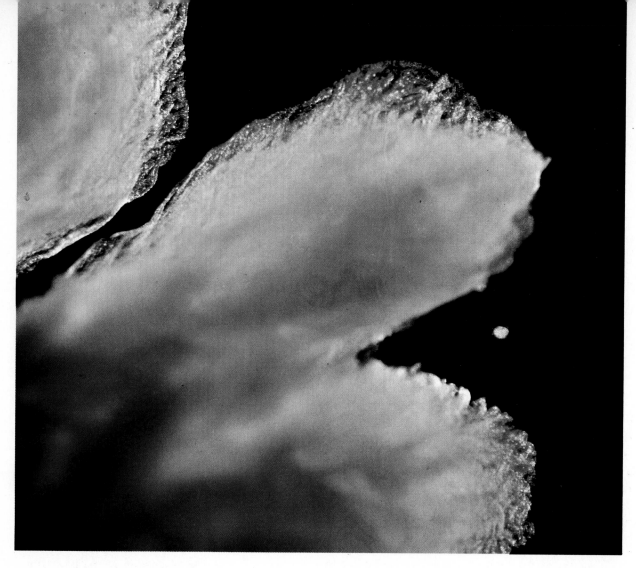

Like a spaceship skirting a solar flare, an ovum is enveloped by the fringes of a Fallopian tube. Beating cilia on the tube's walls create a current that ushers the ovum on its long days' journey to the uterus.

By the cycle's twentieth day, the lining has thickened into a spongy nest copiously endowed with blood vessels and nourishing secretions, awaiting the arrival of a fertilized egg.

Often, the uterus waits in vain. If a fertilized egg nuzzles into the uterine lining, a hormone called human chorionic gonadotropin (HCG) is secreted. HCG resembles LH in chemical structure and strongly mimics its actions. Flowing to the corpus luteum, HCG urges the yellow mass to maintain production of progesterone. But in the absence of fertilization, the corpus luteum lives on borrowed time. It secretes estrogen and progesterone, which halt the pituitary's manufacture of FSH and LH. Deprived of LH, FSH or the chemical substitute HCG, the corpus luteum withers and dies.

The process begins roughly ten days after ovulation. Bereft of HCG, the chemical messenger that announces successful fertilization and implantation, cells in the corpus luteum slow their production of progesterone. Within four or five days, the carefully prepared uterus begins to shed its lining. Arteries that supply the lining constrict, weakening capillary walls. Blood spills from the damaged vessels and detaches layers of the lining, not all at once but in random patches. Endometrium, mucus and blood descend the uterus and then the vagina, creating menstrual flow. The mixture stays fluid because the dying cells of the lining release fibrinolysin, an enzyme that prevents clotting. Menstruation lasts from three to five days, as the uterus sloughs off the thick lining that was three weeks in the making.

Through the ages, human societies have regarded menstruation with a mixture of dread and superstition. The fear and hence the taboo of menstruation is nearly universal. Aristotle believed the glance of a menstruating woman could tarnish a mirror. In sixteenth-century England, menstruating women were forbidden to pickle beef or salt bacon. In his classic study of myth and culture, *The Golden Bough,* Scottish anthropologist Sir James Frazer explored several menstruation taboos. "In Uganda," he noted, "pots which a woman touches while the impurity of menstruation is upon her have to be destroyed; spears and shields defiled by her touch are, however, merely purified." A similar superstition prevails among the Bribri Indians of Costa Rica, who require that menstruating women use banana leaves for plates. After finishing her meal, a woman should throw the leaf in a sequestered place, for a cow that ate the leaf would waste away. In India, many believe that the powers of a menstruating woman can endure beyond her lifetime. One legend maintains that if a woman dies while menstruating, she becomes a malevolent ghost that assumes the form of a beautiful woman who seduces handsome men and spirits them into a private realm. They are returned to the world as gray-haired old men, finding their friends long dead.

The origins of the menstruation taboo are cloaked in mystery. American anthropologist Margaret Mead believed that the superstitions could be traced to primitive man's fear of blood. Whatever its history in folklore, menstruation unquestionably causes many women a healthy measure of both misery and pain. During the monthly flow, these unfortunates — about half the women of childbearing age — complain of agonizing cramps, headaches, back aches and nausea. Scientists have traced the problem to a family of hormonelike chemicals called prostaglandins. Prostaglandins are found in all body cells and influence a host of physiological functions, including the contraction of muscles and constriction of blood vessels. Researchers have shown that prostaglandin levels are four or five times higher in women who experience severe cramps than in those whose menstrual periods are relatively painless. Moreover, plasma drawn from a woman suffering from severe menstrual distress and reinjected into her blood at a later time causes the woman to experience similar symptoms. Today, a variety of drugs are available that counter menstrual pain.

More perplexing than menstrual cramps is the phenomenon called premenstrual syndrome, or PMS. Anywhere from two weeks to a few days before menstruation, many women experience irrational mood swings, headaches, joint pains, weight gain and sore breasts. Occasionally, PMS leads to bizarre behavior. Katharina Dalton, a London family practitioner, recently studied three female convicts and found that their repeated infractions occurred only on days just before their periods. One woman was normally well behaved. At intervals of about twenty-nine days, however, according to Dalton, she would "suddenly burst," attempting arson, assault or even suicide. Eventually, the woman's charge in a fatal stabbing was reduced from murder to manslaughter, because she had committed the crime while in the grip of PMS. Dalton also suspects that Britain's Queen Victoria was a PMS victim. Once a month Victoria would become enraged with her husband Albert, shrieking accusations and throwing objects across the room.

Scientists have not pinpointed the cause of PMS, but strongly suspect that an imbalance in female hormones is the source of the trouble. Dalton has claimed success in treating patients with injections of progesterone ten days before menstruation. Other experts, however, recom-

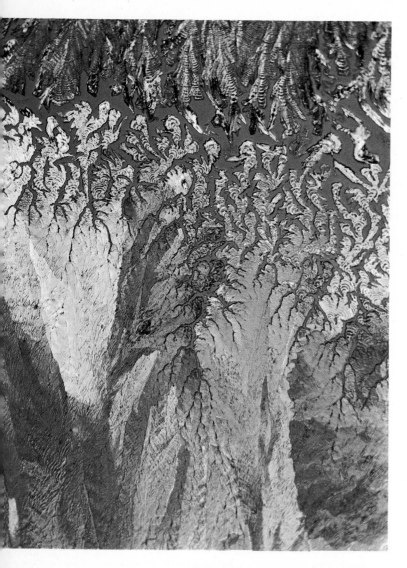

Awakened at puberty, the ovaries secrete estrogen, crystallized above. The hormone causes gradual but profound changes in the female body, including breast growth and widening of the pelvis.

mend diuretics to cut bloating and weight gain and frequent but small high-protein meals to stop precipitous declines in blood sugar, contributing to fatigue and irritability.

Under the orderly timetable of the ovarian cycle, even as menstruation begins, hormones are stimulating the ovaries to initiate a new round of egg development. While the corpus luteum is in full-scale operation, secretions of estrogen and progesterone suppress FSH and LH. While the corpus luteum degenerates, however, dwindling levels of hormone spur fresh surges of FSH and LH, which awaken another fifteen or twenty follicles. Between the ages of forty and fifty, hundreds of follicles have matured, while thousands more have simply degenerated. Overworked ovaries can no longer manufacture estrogen and progesterone, and the menstrual cycle becomes irregular or ceases altogether. The change is called menopause or the climacteric, after the Greek word for "rung of a ladder." Among mammals, women alone lose reproductive powers. Most wild animals never live to advanced age, falling prey to enemies or enfeebled hunting skills. But in zoos, females breed in old age, albeit with less frequency.

Scientists generally agree that declining estrogen production is the key to menopause. They are unsure, however, why some women suffer more unpleasant symptoms than others. One theory proposes that the difficulty lies in how fast estrogen levels drop. Supporters of this hypothesis cite women whose ovaries are surgically removed before menopause. The abrupt halt in estrogen production produces severe menopausal symptoms. Critics of this theory note, however, that if a woman's ovaries are removed before the age of thirty, the symptoms are mild, even though the estrogen drop is equally precipitous. Some researchers suggest that cells become addicted to estrogen. Thus, a lifetime of exposure fosters greater dependency. Withdrawal symptoms result when cells are deprived of the hormone after decades of habituation.

Internally, menopause causes dramatic physical changes. The ovaries shrink and unused eggs and follicles degenerate, to be replaced by fibrous tissue. The Fallopian tubes shed their surface cell layer and shorten. Unneeded for future child-bearing, the uterus shrinks to one-fourth its former size and hardens. The vagina shortens slightly and becomes more narrow. Because its lining gets drier, penetration during intercourse often grows more difficult. Although breasts may atrophy due to glandular shrinking, the change is often offset by new fat deposits.

The outward manifestations of menopause are often more trying. Although some women pass the stage smoothly, many endure a stormy season of headaches, insomnia, itching, weight gain and irritability. Roughly 60 percent feel "hot flashes," warm blushing sensations. More common at night, hot flashes produce heavy sweating. They may last two minutes, and some women must endure them twenty times a day.

Fortunately, treatments are available that counter such menopausal miseries. Some doctors have reported that large doses of vitamin E alleviate hot flashes. Often, estrogen is prescribed to artificially maintain the ovarian cycle, which postpones menopause indefinitely. Although the hormone keeps the body's skin young and the vagina soft, it has been linked with both breast and uterine cancer. The risk of endometrial cancer, particularly serious, is perhaps caused by an abnormal build-up of the uterine lining. The first symptom of endometrial cancer is bleeding, but doctors claim a cure rate of 85 percent if a gynecologist is consulted immediately. Some scientists, however, believe that estrogen may prevent cancer of the ovaries. Ovarian cancer is highly dangerous, because it leaves no warning signs. Some doctors feel that the increased danger of endometrial cancer from taking estrogen is therefore worth the risk, but controversy continues.

Renegade Regeneration

It is a sobering irony that cancer, the abhorred disease marked by the unrestrained reproduction of renegade cells, attacks the reproductive organs of men and women with devastating frequency. Breast cancer is the leading cancer killing women in the United States; more than 100,000 women are struck by the disease each year. Despite this chilling statistic, breast cancer is also easily cured if caught in the early stage, when the tumor is no

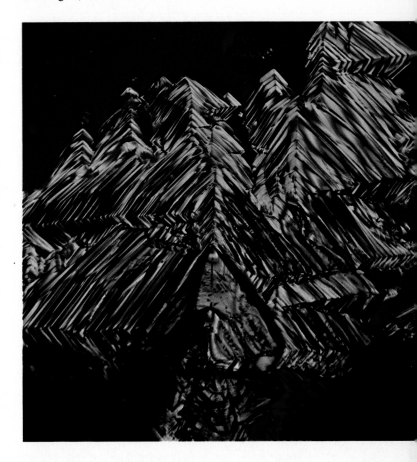

bigger than a marble and has not spread in the body. Eighty to 90 percent of breast cancers detected early are treated successfully.

The cause of breast cancer is still unknown. Nevertheless, scientists suspect that several factors may be involved. Age is clearly important, since most cases occur in women beyond the age of forty. Bearing a child before the age of twenty apparently lowers the risk. Diet may also play a role. In Japan, breast cancer occurs far less frequently than in the United States. Scientists suspect the difference lies in the Japanese diet, which includes less meat and fats. Heredity is also probably a factor. Women with two close relatives who developed breast cancer before menopause stand a fifty-fifty chance themselves. California geneticist Mary-Clair King has studied several generations of families with unusually high rates of breast cancer. In many instances, she and her colleagues found that breast cancer

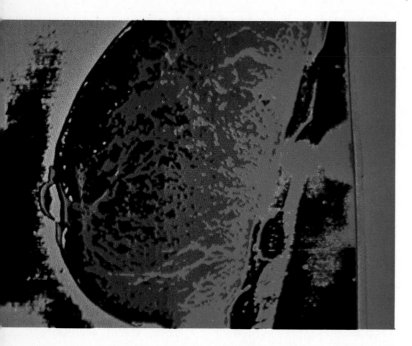

Pincers sunk in flesh, a crablike cancer is revealed by mammograph, an X-ray of the breast. Both Greeks and Romans noted the resemblance, naming the disease after the Greek for "crab." Breast cancer strikes 100,000 American women each year. Detected early, it is often curable. Doctors have traditionally treated the cancer with mastectomy, but research shows that less drastic measures can be equally effective.

was associated with the presence of a particular enzyme. The researchers believe that the breast cancers in these families are caused by a gene linked to the enzyme-producing gene.

The early detection of breast cancer rests on women regularly examining their breasts. They should check once every month in the week after menstrual flow stops. Women who are not menstruating, whether they are past menopause, pregnant or nursing, should check on the first day of the month. Danger signs include changes in the projecting angle of the nipple, dimples, variations in the size of the areola and internal lumps. Sixty to 80 percent of such lumps are harmless, but only a doctor should make this determination. Harmless lumps — milk glands, fat lobules and benign cysts — are generally smooth and movable. Cancerous lumps are hard and rough, because they reach into adjacent tissue like the claws of a crab. The resemblance was noted long ago by Hippocrates, who named the disease *karkinoma,* meaning "crab." Unusual nipple secretions may also spell danger. Secretions are common, especially during or soon after pregnancy. But women should be wary of secretions that flow without forceful squeezing from a single pore in the nipple of one breast.

Doctors can now mobilize a battery of diagnostic weapons to find tumors. Mammography, an offshoot of the conventional X-ray, reveals the breast's internal structure, including glands, blood vessels and muscles. Clots, cysts and tumors show up as dark spots. A new generation of devices, using the technology of office copying machines, produces instant pictures of high resolution. Concerns over radiation hazards have spurred the development of other diagnostic methods, such as ultrasound, a technique based on the principles of sonar.

Doctors have traditionally treated breast tumors with mastectomy, the surgical amputation of the breast. The procedure has long been used. An Egyptian medical papyrus written around 1500 B.C. recommends healing fatty tumors "with the knife." The Roman physician Galen claimed the cause of most cancers was excess bile and he prescribed special diets for treatment. For breast cancer, however, he advocated surgery. In the seventeenth century, Italian surgeon Marcus Aurelius Severino recommended the removal of enlarged lymph nodes along with the breast. By 1889, Baltimore surgeon William Halstead had refined the procedure, performing radical mastectomies that removed layers of chest muscle and lymph nodes under the arm. Today, doctors have drastically cut death by breast cancer through mastectomy. Recent studies indicate, however, that the disfiguring procedure may be unnecessary in many cases. Simple excision of the lump, along with radiation therapy, is often equally effective if the cancer is detected early.

Cancer of the cervix is less widespread than breast cancer, but just as dangerous. Although nearly 6,000 American women were killed by the disease in 1978, deaths have fallen dramatically in recent years. Doctors attribute this small victory to the Pap smear, a simple test of cervical cells that reliably reports the presence of cancer. Sexually active women are probably at greater risk, because scientists now think cervical cancer behaves like a venereal disease, in that it is transmitted through sexual intercourse. Studies have shown that nuns never develop it, while prostitutes are afflicted frequently. Women whose sexual partners have had vasectomies run a lower

George Nicholas Papanicolaou

A Greek Bearing Cures

"Only the weak and cowardly seek harbors," declared George Papanicolaou, then twenty-one years old, to his father in 1904. "It is better for me to be destroyed, erased, than to have my soul say, 'Wait! Enough of dreaming.'" Just nine years later, Papanicolaou's dreams carried him from his Greek homeland to New York harbor, seeking opportunities in medical research. The voyage was fruitful for Papanicolaou and his adopted country. In 1925, he discovered a reliable method of detecting cervical cancer in its early stages, when it can still be treated. Before he died in 1962, Papanicolaou saw the death rate from cervical cancer cut nearly 50 percent, largely due to his simple procedure — the Pap test.

Born on the Greek island of Euboea, Papanicolaou attended medical school in Athens. Pressed by his father to become a military physician, he rebelled against the idea, preferring a career in research. For a brief spell, he practiced medicine in his hometown, treating among others the residents of a nearby leper colony. Starved for intellectual challenge, he entered Germany's University of Jena in 1907 to study zoology. Four years later, he helped analyze marine specimens aboard a research

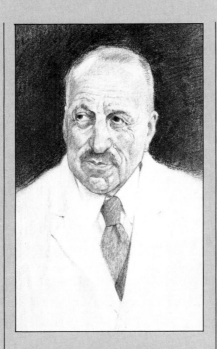

vessel built and captained by Prince Albert I of Monaco. The expedition spent two weeks off the shores of Madeira and the Canary Islands, and caught a whale near the Azores which Papanicolaou dissected. The following year, he served as a doctor in the Greek army during a war against Turkey which lasted but seven months before a peace treaty was concluded in London.

Finding conditions in Greece "unfavorable to the continuation of biological research" due to inadequate laboratory facilities, Papanicolaou embarked for America. While his wife sewed buttons on clothes for five dollars a week, he found a job selling rugs at Gimbel's department store. On his second day at work, however, a woman he had met on his passage to America came to the store as a customer. Ashamed to be seen selling rugs, he appealed to a scientist acquaintance to find him a research position. He soon found work at the Cornell Medical School. He remained and eventually became a professor.

In the 1920s, Papanicolaou began studying smears from the vagina. Unexpectedly, he found that cancer cells could sometimes be observed, a discovery he later called among the "most thrilling" of his career. Initially, Papanicolaou's medical colleagues were skeptical of his findings, preferring to use biopsies after cancerous lesions could be seen on the cervix. Undeterred, he pressed on, finding that vaginal smears revealed cancer at its early stages, before any lesion appeared. Improved methods of staining which he later developed made the renegade cells more clearly visible. In 1948, the American Cancer Society concluded that vaginal smears were indispensable to the early detection of cervical cancer. Within a few years, the Pap test became a stock weapon in the war on cancer.

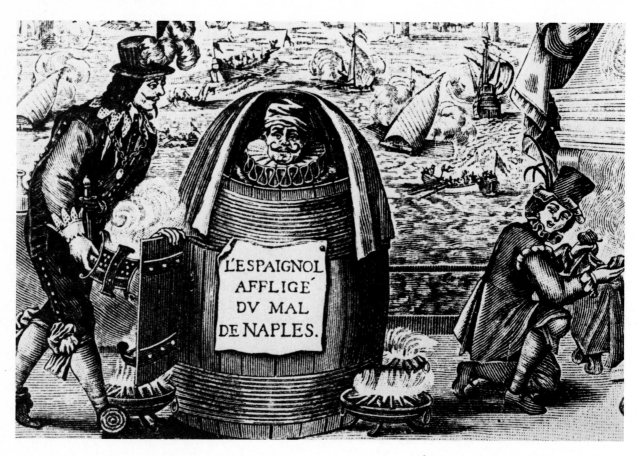

risk of cervical cancer, leading some scientists to suspect that sperm might carry a cancer virus.

Among men, the leading fatal cancer is cancer of the prostate, a gland that contributes fluids to semen. Each year, prostate cancer claims 17,000 victims in the United States alone. Older men have traces of the disease in overwhelming numbers. Autopsies of men who have died of causes other than cancer reveal that 30 percent of all men in their sixties have some degree of prostate cancer. For men in their eighties, the figure rises to more than 80 percent. Generally, however, the cancer is slow to progress. Men in their eighties are far more likely to succumb to heart disease.

Early cancer of the prostate has no symptoms. By the time doctors can detect the disease, in half of all cases it has spread throughout the body. If the cancer is confined to the prostate, doctors surgically remove the gland, which often creates problems in urinary control. But even if the can-

cer has spread, hope remains. In 1941, Canadian-born urologist Charles Huggins discovered that prostate cancer, no matter how widespread, is dependent on testosterone for continued growth. When testosterone production is shut down, through castration, the cancer often disappears. The reversal can be almost magical. Reproductive biologist and microsurgeon Sherman Silber has remarked, "Patients who appeared to be on their deathbed, in miserable pain, and nearly comatose," improved "overnight" after surgery and were ready to "go home within the week."

Cancer also strikes the testicles. Testicular cancer is rare, but on the rise. In the past forty years, the incidence has doubled. Four thousand new cases are diagnosed each year. It is now the most common cancer in men between the ages of twenty and thirty-four. For unknown reasons, the disease strikes white middle- and upper-class men most frequently. If detected early, it can

60

usually be cured. Doctors recommend that men regularly check their testicles, preferably in a warm shower when the scrotum is relaxed, for small lumps the size of a pea.

The Great Pox

"Love's a capricious power," wrote Byron in *Don Juan*. Perhaps nowhere is that power displayed more capriciously than in the scourge of venereal disease. Probably the most notorious is syphilis, a contagion caused by bacteria called spirochetes, which can infiltrate the body wherever they find an opening. Dentists have contracted syphilis when spirochetes in a patient's mouth invaded a cut in the dentist's finger. Such cases, however, are generally flukes. In almost every instance, the spirochetes are transmitted through sexual contact, either oral or genital.

Syphilis first appeared in Europe at the close of the fifteenth century, and many scholars believe that the disease was carried by sailors returning with Columbus from America. The first recorded epidemic broke out in Naples in 1495. Some of the sailors may have joined the army of Charles VIII of France, who was laying siege to the city. Later commenting on the disease, French philosopher Voltaire wryly noted that "when the French dashed headlong into Italy, they easily won Naples and the pox; then they were driven out, but they did not lose everything, for they took the pox with them." Syphilis spread across Europe rapidly. In seeking to explain the new disease, German Emperor Maximilian issued a pamphlet in 1495 proclaiming that God had sent syphilis as a punishment for blasphemy. The following year, an official in Nuremberg published another pamphlet, illustrated by Albrecht Dürer, declaring that bad positioning of the planets was to blame. English history was irrevocably altered by syphilis when Henry VIII caught the disease around 1510, within a year of his marriage to Catharine of Aragon, his first wife. Catharine bore four sons before 1515, all stillborn or fatally infected with syphilis. Desperate for a male heir, Henry petitioned Pope Clement VII to annul his marriage. After several years of bitter feuding, and the Pope's ultimate refusal to annul the marriage, Henry broke with the Catholic Church.

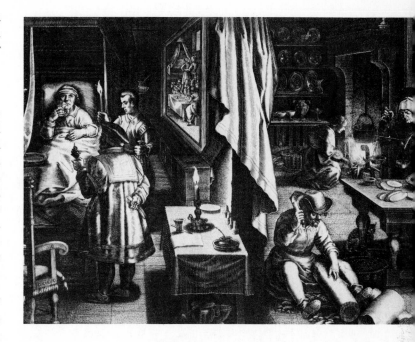

Syphilis sufferers of the 1500s drank a broth made from guaiacum, a tropical New World tree. Briefly touted as a miracle cure for syphilis, guaiacum offered little relief for those wasted by the disease.

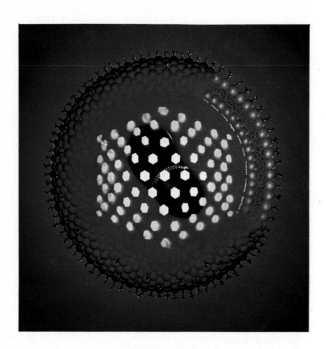

A menacing alien world, the herpes simplex II virus erupts in sores around the genitals. Researchers believe the epidemic venereal disease infects perhaps twenty million Americans. No cure is yet known, but scientists are exploring several avenues of treatment, including vaccines. The government recently approved the commercial distribution of an ointment containing acyclovir, a drug to alleviate herpes symptoms.

Syphilis owes its insidious power to biological mechanisms that mask its symptoms. Then, years after its outward signs have vanished, the disease reappears, like a recurring nightmare. The first warning of syphilis is a chancre, or sore, which afflicts the genitals ten to ninety days after the initial infection. Within a few weeks, the chancre heals, but the disease has only gone underground. About a month later, new symptoms emerge. They usually include rashes, headaches and the shedding of hair in patches. Again, symptoms disappear within weeks. The final stage begins two to five years later. Although the victim may feel healthy, the deadly spirochetes can cause irreversible heart and brain damage over the following twenty years. British political leader Randolph Churchill, Winston's father, died after syphilis had slowly destroyed his once brilliant mind. Today, doctors immediately prescribe penicillin to fight syphilis. The antibiotic drug is extraordinarily effective, usually bringing about complete cures.

Gonorrhea, another venereal disease, has a less colorful history than syphilis, but perhaps greater antiquity. Roman physician Galen named the disease but, because its symptoms are less devastating, it was overshadowed by syphilis after 1500. In men, the gonorrhea germ causes a drip from the penis, often accompanied by pain during urination, around three to six days after infection. Eighty percent of women infected with gonorrhea feel no symptoms, but they may feel a burning sensation during urination. Untreated, gonorrhea may cause sterility, arthritis and heart trouble. Statistics add an ominous dimension to such dangers, since two million Americans contract the disease each year. Fortunately, like syphilis, gonorrhea is easily cured by antibiotics. But doctors are concerned by the emergence of a new strain of gonorrhea that is resistant to penicillin. They think it was probably imported to the United States by servicemen returning from the Philippines. Although another antibiotic is being used to kill it, the strain could develop even hardier resistance. Should that happen, scientists fear a medical disaster.

Alongside these older contagions, a new venereal disease, herpes, has infected up to twenty million Americans. Unlike syphilis and gonorrhea, herpes is incurable. The herpes viruses cause chicken pox, mononucleosis and other ailments. One branch of the viral family, herpes simplex II, produces painful blisters on or near the genitals several days after intercourse with an infected partner. The sores are generally accompanied by fever and muscle aches. After a few weeks, the virus goes into hibernation in nerve cells at the base of the spine, and its symptoms disappear. In some victims, the symptoms never return. Others must endure fresh attacks by the virus every month.

Herpes is most contagious during such outbreaks, but people with mild cases can transmit the disease unknowingly. Pregnant women are at greater risk, because they can transmit the virus to their babies during delivery. Most infected babies suffer blindness or brain damage. Some die. Women infected by herpes also run a higher risk of developing cervical cancer. Although scientists are vigorously exploring potential cures for the disease, success remains elusive.

A Primal Force

Microorganisms that attack man through sex have chosen a sure avenue for survival, for man has always enthusiastically obeyed the biblical injunction to "Be fruitful, and multiply, and replenish the earth." In sex, man is driven by a primal force that poet Walt Whitman called "the procreant urge of the world." By canny design, Nature has made sex deeply pleasurable, an irresistible tide carrying new generations on its crest.

In men, sexual excitement begins with erection of the penis. Nerve impulses jump from the brain to the sacral cord, a section of five fused vertebrae in the lower spine, where an erection center is housed. In turn, signals from the sacral cord stimulate nerves that dilate arteries leading to the penis. Blood quickly fills three tubes of spongy tissue in the penis, causing them to swell. Erectile tissue presses against veins in the penis, slowing the exit of blood.

Shifting patterns of blood flow also play a crucial role in a woman's sexual response. During arousal, tissues around the vagina fill with blood. Sex researchers Virginia Johnson and William

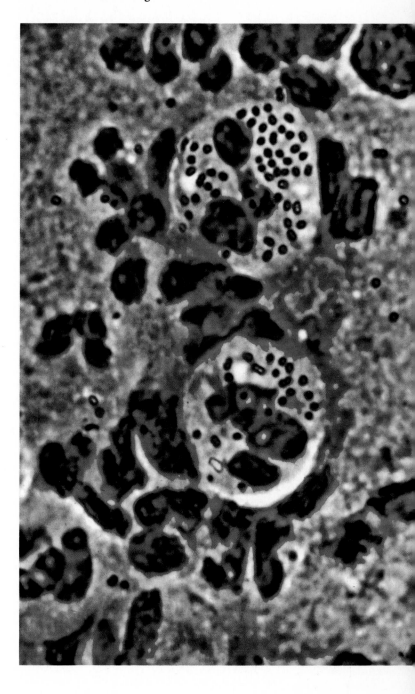

Masters have found that beads of lubricant form on the vaginal walls like beads of sweat. Besides easing penetration during intercourse, vaginal secretions have another role in reproduction. The vagina normally has an acidic environment, only marginally hospitable to sperm. Because the secretions are slightly alkaline, they reduce acidity, thus enhancing the prospect that sperm will survive to reach the egg. Arousal also causes blood to engorge the clitoris and nipples. Internally, the vagina expands, like an inflated balloon. The uterus draws away from the vagina as sexual excitement increases.

In recent years, scientists have embarked on an exhaustive search for chemicals known as pheromones in vaginal secretions. In many animals, pheromones attract sexual partners. Paper doused in bombykol, a substance secreted by female silkworm moths, lures male moths. In 1970, researchers at the Georgia Mental Health Institute reported from experiments with rhesus monkeys that vaginal chemicals called copulins appeared to excite the males. Subsequent investigations cast doubt on these findings, but some scientists maintain that copulins, also found in women's vaginal secretions, play some role in human sexuality. In 1980, British scientists announced the discovery of a chemical in men's sweat which they believe is a pheromone. The substance smells like sandalwood oil, often used in perfumes. Scientists are also baffled by experiments showing that human sexual activity increases at the time of ovulation, a phenomenon possibly caused by pheromones. Despite such tantalizing clues, however, many scientists remain skeptical about the existence of human pheromones, and the search continues.

Among animals, the sex act is usually brief. Bulls and rams ejaculate within a few seconds, as do lions and chimpanzees. In dogs and wolves, copulation may last longer. Human intercourse varies in duration. One survey of American couples revealed that 75 percent completed sex within ten minutes. Mae West reported in her autobiography that one man made love to her for fifteen hours, a possible record. Such feats of sexual endurance, however, are difficult to sustain. Nerve impulses from the penis travel to the cerebral cortex. As the intensity of stimuli builds, reflex centers in the spinal cord send impulses to the genitals, prompting a process called emission. First, contractions of smooth muscles on the testicles, epididymes and vasa deferentia force sperm into the urethra. There, any traces of urine —acidic and lethal to sperm — in the urethra have already been neutralized by secretions from Cowper's glands, two pea-sized organs below the prostate. The prostate gland and seminal vesicles then add their contributions to the mixture, pushing the sperm forward in the urethra. Fluid from the prostate adds bulk to the semen and neutralizes acid secretions from the vagina, as well as the carbonic acid in the vas deferens that keeps sperm in suspended animation.

After emission, a man no longer exerts voluntary control over ejaculation. The filling of the urethra with mixed glandular fluids and sperm sends a new message to the spinal cord, which reacts by transmitting impulses to muscles that encase the base of the penis. The muscles contract, forcing semen out under great pressure. A vast flotilla of sperm, perhaps 500 million strong, has been launched to besiege the solitary egg waiting in the Fallopian tube.

The Moment of Union

Inside the vagina, events proceed apace. Roused from their slumber, the sperm swim by lashing their tails, moving about half an inch per minute. At the leading edge of the seminal assault, citric acid helps dissolve the mucous plug sealing the cervix and blocking entry to the uterus. The process is abetted by prostaglandins contributed by the seminal vesicles. Prostaglandins may also cause contractions in the uterus and Fallopian tubes, sucking sperm toward the egg. Some scientists believe that the female orgasm performs the same function. The seminal vesicles also add fructose to the semen, to nourish the sperm during their journey.

Of the hundreds of millions of sperm that are ejaculated only tens of thousands gain access to the uterus through the portal of the cervix. The rest are left behind in the vagina. Inside the womb, sperm find a welcome environment rich in glucose, which fires them into a new burst of

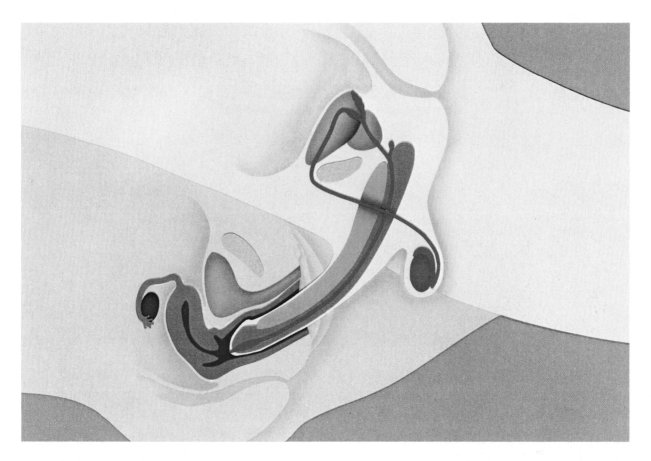

energy. The fastest sperm take the lead and travel up the Fallopian tubes, like salmon migrating to their spawning grounds. Usually, only one tube harbors an egg, but a readied ovum can lie in both. If both ova are fertilized, the womb will shelter fraternal twins. Likewise, one ovary can sometimes ripen two ova, releasing them into a single Fallopian tube. Again, fraternal twins may develop if both eggs are fertilized.

The first sperm that reach the egg dash headlong against it, in an almost frantic effort to penetrate. Each sperm is tipped with an acrosome, a percussion cap that opens to release an enzyme called hyaluronidase. Like a chemical knife, hyaluronidase slices through the chemical coating of the egg, clearing a trail for the sperm.

Although many sperm are wriggling against the egg, only one gains the upper hand, much like a sprinter who is a pace ahead at the final tape. Aided by its enzyme machete, this sperm

Powerful muscle contractions in the penis cause ejaculation, the discharge of semen into the vagina. Of the perhaps 500 million sperm launched, only one will penetrate an ovum, creating an embryo.

Overrun with sperm, a sea urchin's egg awaits fertilization, below left. Scientists have extensively studied fertilization in marine invertebrates because they release eggs and sperm in sea water, making the process *easy to duplicate in the laboratory. The mechanics of human fertilization are similar. When a sperm strikes, below right, its tip opens like a percussion cap, releasing an enzyme to dissolve the egg's surface.*

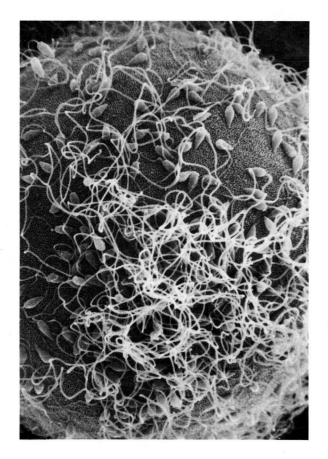

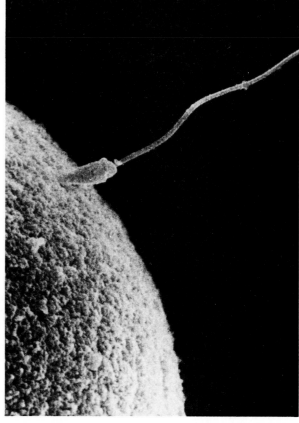

manages to penetrate the egg. Quickly, the egg's surface changes to block the entry of other sperm. Within seconds, electrical shifts resembling a nerve impulse apparently act as a preliminary barrier. Then, as the chosen sperm penetrates the egg, thousands of small sacs just beneath the egg's surface discharge enzymes. One alters receptor sites on the egg, detaching sperm already bound to the surface and preventing others from binding. The other enzyme allows the outer surface to separate from deeper layers, creating an impassable barrier.

Once a sperm has entered, the egg begins further preparations for the uniting of their genetic material. When it left the ovary, the egg contained forty-six chromosomes, the normal number in a human cell. At fertilization, a second division occurs through meiosis. The egg halves its chromosomes to twenty-three, casting out another polar body. When the sperm reaches the egg's deepest interior, its twenty-three chromosomes meet the egg's. For a moment, they hesitate. Then, the chromosomes neatly pair off. In nine months, the solitary new cell will have grown into a human being.

On the chromosome strands of the fertilized egg are coils of deoxyribonucleic acid (DNA), arranged into units called genes. Encoded on genes is the blueprint for human traits, from eye color to the shape of feet. Scientists do not know how many genes are in a single human cell, but the estimates range from 100,000 to half a million. Curiously, the cell apparently harbors far more DNA than is needed to sustain life. Nor is this puzzling characteristic unique to man. The Easter lily has ten times as much DNA as man. The African lungfish, an odd variety equipped with both gills and lungs, has forty-two times as much DNA, cell for cell, as man. Biologist Francis Crick, who won a Nobel prize for helping to un-

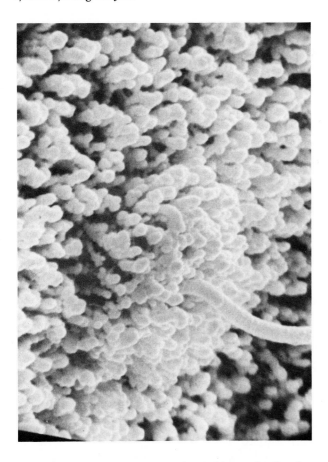

chromosomes in women, and one X- and one Y-shaped chromosome in men. At fertilization, the female egg keeps one of its X chromosomes. But in the process of sperm formation in the testicles, each sperm gets either an X or Y. The joining of an X sperm with the egg creates a female embryo. Fertilization by a Y sperm creates a male.

The Ratio Evened

Because X and Y sperm are manufactured in equal number, mathematical odds would seem to dictate equal numbers of men and women. But statistics reveal that 106 boys are born for every 100 girls. Scientists speculate that Y sperm swim faster than their X counterparts, perhaps because the X sperm carry slightly more genetic material and are bogged down. As a result, Y sperm are more likely to reach the egg first. Nevertheless, Nature seems to have a plan behind the uneven numbers. Contrary to popular belief, women are biologically hardier than men, who perish at a higher rate. Between the ages of fourteen to eighteen, when the reproductive years begin, the male to female ratio is even.

Sometimes, the distribution of the sex chromosomes is skewed, resulting in babies with genetic abnormalities. One woman in six thousand is afflicted with Turner's syndrome, a condition caused by the absence of one X chromosome. As adults, women with Turner's syndrome are shorter than average but have normal intelligence. Because their ovaries are undeveloped, they need hormone therapy to artificially induce breast development and menstrual periods.

Occasionally, sperm carry two Y chromosomes. For many years, a myth persisted that the XYY males had criminal tendencies. Recent research, however, has proved the concept untrue. John Money, professor of medical psychology and pediatrics at Johns Hopkins University, says that many XYY males "really suffer." They "impulsively cry, panic, attack, laugh or even commit suicide by jumping off a bridge, as one of my patients did." Yet, other XYY men show no such problems. Scientists remain puzzled why some are irrationally impulsive while others are not.

Although XYY males and victims of Turner's syndrome are relatively rare, genetic defects are

ravel the molecular structure of DNA, thinks the excess DNA thrives within a cell like "a not too harmful parasite within its host." Crick's hypothesis builds on the controversial idea, prominently espoused by British sociobiologist Richard Dawkins, that living creatures are simply efficient machines designed to perpetuate genes.

Among the genes that earn their keep are those that determine whether an embryo will become a man or a woman. The Japanese of the tenth century believed that if a pregnant woman concentrated on male activities, like hunting, she would have a boy. In eighteenth-century France, some noblemen were advised by physicians that removal of the left testicle would assure a male heir. Both notions were wrong, but the French were slightly closer to the truth, for sex is determined by genes carried by the man. In humans, chromosomes come in pairs, twenty-three in all. The twenty-third pair consists of two X-shaped

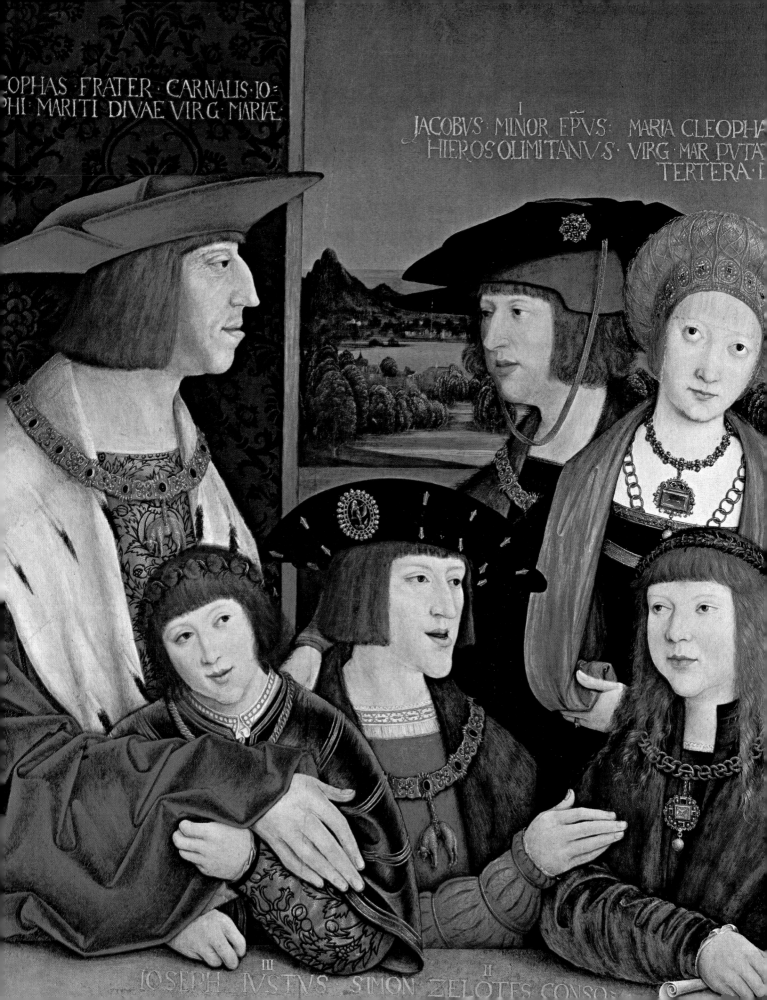

OPHAS FRATER CARNALIS IO=
PHI MARITI DIVAE VIRG MARIAE

JACOBVS MINOR EPVS
HIEROSOLIMITANVS

MARIA CLEOPHA
VIRG MAR PVTA
TERTERA

IOSEPH IVSTVS   SIMON ZELOTES CONSO

universal. Each person carries anywhere from
four to eight defective genes. Because these genes
run in families, intermarriage between relatives
greatly increases the risk of birth defects. Studies
of isolated communities in Martha's Vineyard,
the Kentucky mountains, Sweden and Japan,
where intermarriage is common, have shown a
high incidence of deafness, dwarfism, albinism or
feeble-mindedness. Scientists have identified
nearly 3,000 genetically transmitted diseases,
1,300 of them since 1966.

Many genetic disorders center on the body's
inability to manufacture a particular enzyme. In
Fabry's disease, the enzyme needed to break
down a fatty substance is missing. The defect
leads to high blood pressure, kidney failure and
strokes. Another enzyme-related disease, Lesch-
Nyhan syndrome, leads to bizarre behavior, including self-mutilation. Some patients manifest
this symptom by severely biting themselves
around the mouth and limbs.

Huntington's chorea is a rare hereditary disease that strikes the nervous system, leading to
mental and physical decline. The name derives
from *choreia*, Greek for "dance," because the disease's victims wave their limbs in aimless mo-
tions. More than a thousand cases in the United
States have been traced to three brothers who
arrived from England in colonial times. The disease is especially pernicious because symptoms
are hidden until middle age. People with an affected parent endure years of uncertainty before
learning whether they have inherited the gene.

Songwriter Woody Guthrie, a prominent victim of Huntington's chorea, spent nearly fifteen
years as a hospitalized invalid before succumbing
in 1967. In his autobiography, *Bound for Glory*,
Guthrie described his mother's tragic decline,
then attributed to insanity. Now Guthrie's son
Arlo, himself a successful musician, is approaching middle age, and will soon learn whether he
shares his father's unhappy fate. Fortunately,
most genetic diseases, like Huntington's chorea,
are rare. At fertilization, the genetic blueprint, for
better or worse, is fixed. Over the next nine
months, the fertilized egg, a speck barely visible
to the naked eye, will fulfill its unique genetic
destiny — to become a human being.

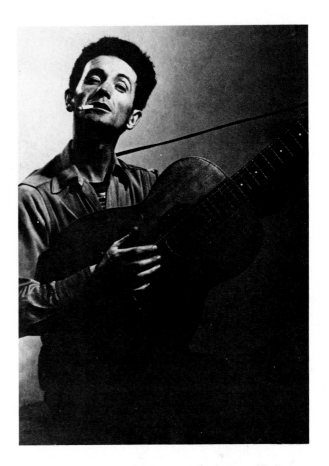

Champion of the downtrodden,
Oklahoma songwriter Woody
Guthrie was felled by Huntington's
chorea, a genetic disease that strikes
in middle age and leads to gradual
degeneration of the nervous system.

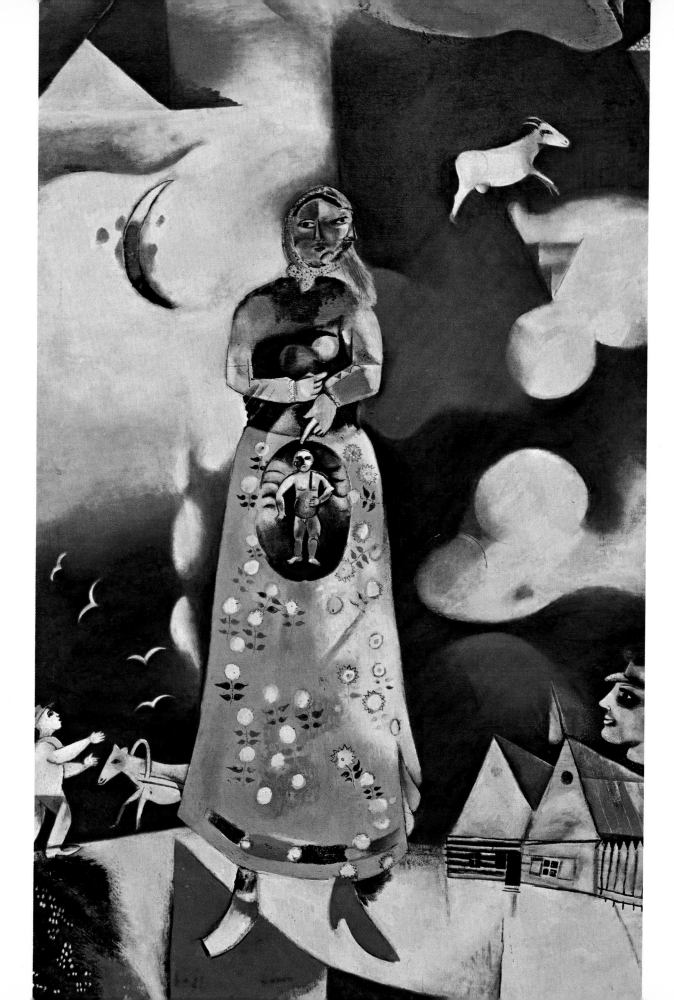

Chapter 3

A Sudden Quickening

The history of a man for the nine months preceding his birth would, probably, be far more interesting and contain events of greater moment than all the three score and ten years that follow it," mused English poet Samuel Taylor Coleridge in 1802. Beginning with a single cell smaller than the dot above this "i," this history closes with a child of some 200 billion cells, stretching about twenty inches from head to foot and weighing around seven pounds. Never again in life does a person grow so rapidly or develop so diversely. Between conception and birth, cells multiply, change and place themselves in patterns that shape a distinct human form.

Long ago Aristotle observed that "He who sees things grow from the beginning will have the finest view of them." As archaeology records the beginnings of civilization, so embryology writes the biography of an unborn child. "Biographies," Mark Twain reckoned, "are but the clothes and buttons of the man." Today, in a time that one Harvard scientist calls "the most exciting period of developmental biology since the turn of the century," embryologists are finding that the unborn dress in strange and marvelous attire.

Within hours of conception the fertilized egg, a zygote, begins to grow and develop. Formed in the upper reaches of the Fallopian tube, it drifts down toward the uterus on a current stirred by flutterings of fine hairs, the cilia, lining the tube. Muscular contractions of the tube itself ensure the zygote's journey. As it tumbles downstream it divides into like cells — first two, then four, eight, sixteen and so on.

To divide, the zygote must be awash in progesterone, one of two major female hormones. Early in pregnancy, the hormone is secreted by the corpus luteum, a yellow mass of cells formed in the empty follicle abandoned by the mature ovum. Division is spurred as deoxyribonucleic acid (DNA) reproduces itself, generating the proteins

Memory bears civilization as a mother carries life. In Maternité, *composed in 1913, Marc Chagall paints an expectant mother against a background of impressions recalled from his childhood in rural Russia. Pointing to her womb, opened like a window, the woman proclaims the child to come. Behind her, scenes tell of the world the child will enter.*

that enliven the cells. Three days after fertilization, the eight-celled zygote contains more than a thousand different proteins. Their quantity, but not variety, will increase as division continues.

Around the fourth day the zygote, comprising some sixteen cells, enters the uterus where it floats freely for a day or so. As it continues to grow, the cells ready themselves for different roles. A cavity opens amid the dividing cells, changing the zygote into a hollow ball called a blastocyst. At the same time, cells distinguish themselves from one another. Most flatten out to form the outer cell mass, or trophoblast, a strand of single cells ringing the blastocyst. In time, the trophoblast will produce the placenta, source of nourishment for the growing fetus. The remaining cells cluster together at one end of the cavity to make the inner cell mass, the embryoblast, from which embryo, fetus and child will emerge. Both placenta and fetus arise from this same single cell — the zygote.

A Time to Plant

Once the blastocyst is formed, the trophoblast prods the mother into making the arrangements necessary for embedding it in the endometrium, the wall of the uterus. This, too, is the task of hormones. Along with progesterone, the hormone estrogen readies the mother's uterine wall to receive the blastocyst. On its second day in the womb, the blastocyst nuzzles up to the endometrium, already made soft and porous by progesterone and estrogen.

The blastocyst implants itself in the wall of the uterus, readied by hormones, in a process that takes about a week to complete. Quivering villi from the trophoblast and the endometrium reach toward each other, gently caress, then tightly embrace to forge the first bond between mother and offspring. Meanwhile, the trophoblast splits in two. One part, the syncytiotrophoblast, burrows aggressively into the endometrium, devouring tissue to hollow out a nest. As it moves through the endometrium, it dredges small pools which soon fill with blood from the mother's circulation. Behind this advancing cutting edge, the second part, the cytotrophoblast, sprouts a web of primary villi, which reach through to the pools

of maternal blood. By the fifteenth day or so, the primary villi are heavily laced with blood vessels. The blood vessels run through tissue called the body stalk, stretched like a causeway between the trophoblast and embryoblast, that later becomes the umbilical cord. With the tapping of the maternal blood stream, primitive circulation between mother and embryo begins. Like a plant sinking roots in soil, the placenta begins to grow.

After implantation, tiny projections called chorionic villi extend from the trophoblast to secrete a third hormone, human chorionic gonadotropin (HCG). HCG sustains the life of the corpus luteum, perpetuating its secretion of hormones without which the pregnancy would be thwarted.

When the zygote implants itself somewhere other than the uterus the pregnancy is said to be ectopic. Ectopic pregnancies occur once in every 125 to 300 cases, more often among nonwhites than whites and among poor than well-to-do women. In 95 percent of all ectopic pregnancies, the zygote implants itself in the Fallopian tube. Diagnosis may prove elusive, especially if the tube does not rupture to cause severe abdominal pain and bleeding. Such pregnancies are terminated by a surgical procedure suited to the pregnancy's location and the patient's condition as well as her intentions of future childbearing.

At the same time, other cells from the trophoblast form a membrane called the chorion, which surrounds all the structures arisen from the fertilized egg. The chorion lines the chamber within the uterine wall housing the developing embryo and placenta. Soon, during the second week, the amniotic cavity, ringed by another membrane, the amnion, forms inside the chorion's chamber to provide the inner sanctum for the embryo.

While the trophoblast spearheads implantation, the embryoblast develops in its train. About midway through implantation the embryoblast differentiates into two adjoining layers of cells. The ectoderm, the outside layer, is composed of tall columnar cells. The inner layer is the endoderm, made of small, individual cube-shaped cells. Together they form what scientists call the embryonic disk. Early in the third week, the disk grows and lengthens, taking on a pearlike shape. A fissure, called the primitive streak, forms in the

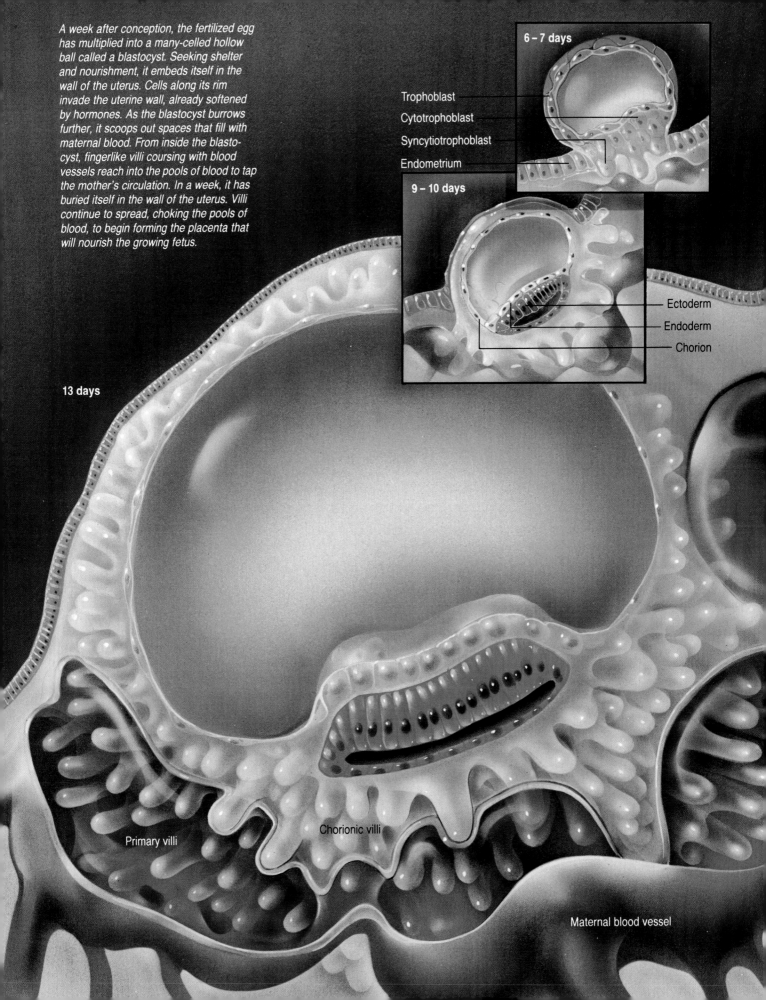

A week after conception, the fertilized egg has multiplied into a many-celled hollow ball called a blastocyst. Seeking shelter and nourishment, it embeds itself in the wall of the uterus. Cells along its rim invade the uterine wall, already softened by hormones. As the blastocyst burrows further, it scoops out spaces that fill with maternal blood. From inside the blasto-cyst, fingerlike villi coursing with blood vessels reach into the pools of blood to tap the mother's circulation. In a week, it has buried itself in the wall of the uterus. Villi continue to spread, choking the pools of blood, to begin forming the placenta that will nourish the growing fetus.

6 – 7 days

Trophoblast
Cytotrophoblast
Syncytiotrophoblast
Endometrium

9 – 10 days

Ectoderm
Endoderm
Chorion

13 days

Primary villi

Chorionic villi

Maternal blood vessel

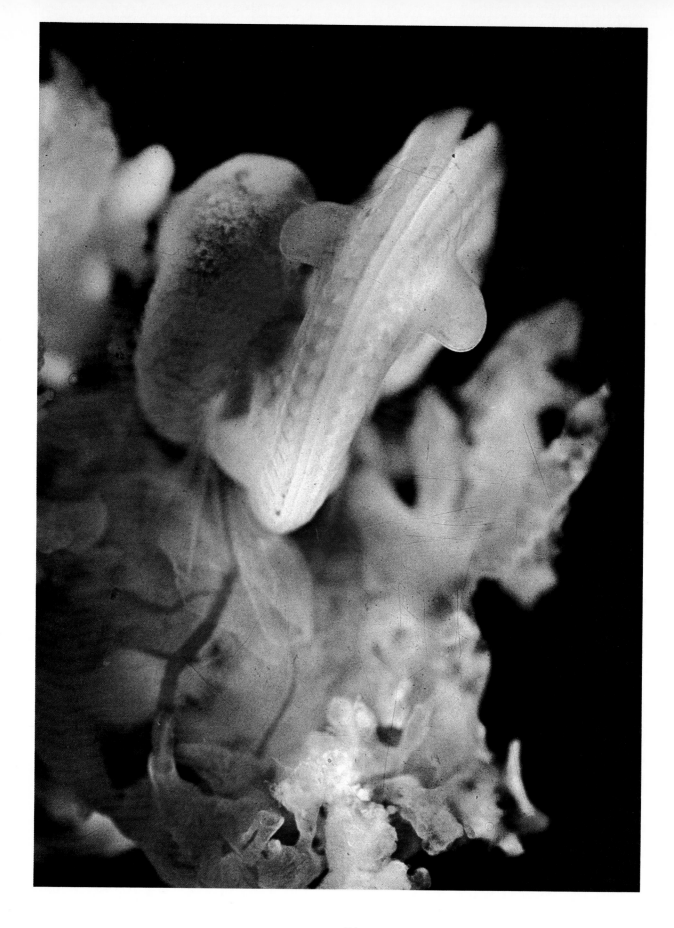

ectoderm along the length of the embryo. The ectoderm's cells edge toward the fissure, slip into it and spread sideways to form a third layer of cells, the mesoderm, between the other two. Each of the three layers will produce particular tissues, organs and systems.

By now the mother has begun to suspect her pregnancy. Normally, menstruation would begin on the first day of the third week after conception. Even before she misses her first period, her suspicions may be aroused by signs sometimes mistaken for harbingers of menstruation. Her breasts grow full and tender, especially at the nipples. She suffers nausea, the traditional "morning sickness," either with or without vomiting. Pressure of the swelling uterus on her bladder prompts her to urinate more often. Tiring easily, she may feel listless and lethargic and perhaps unusually moody or tearful.

Her suspicions heightened by her failure to menstruate, the woman visits a physician who can most likely confirm the pregnancy by internal examination. A softening of the lower uterus, caused by its engorgement with blood, can be detected a week or two after the missed period. A little later, heavier blood flow to pelvic organs may lend a bluish hue to the cervix or vagina. Although more reliable than the evidence interpreted by the mother herself, these signs do not necessarily occur in all women or they may arise from other causes.

So physicians check their diagnoses against one of several pregnancy tests. All pregnancy tests measure levels of HCG in either blood or urine samples. The level of HCG rises throughout the first seventy days of pregnancy. Some blood tests are so sensitive they register HCG within a week of fertilization. But tests given ten to fourteen days after the first missed period yield the most reliable results.

Since 1976, kits for performing pregnancy tests at home have been marketed in drugstores and supermarkets. Although the tests offer privacy and convenience, their accuracy has been challenged. Studies have found the tests 97 percent accurate for women who were pregnant, but only 80 percent accurate for those who were not. The manufacturers, conceding this shortcoming, rec-

ommend that women who get a negative result repeat the test a week later. The accuracy of the test depends on its proper conduct and interpretation, says one nurse-practitioner who regularly cares for pregnant women. "In seeking the answer to such an important question," she adds, "why not rely on those best qualified to give it?"

The confirmed pregnancy heralds an onrush of change, for over the next five weeks the embryo undergoes its most dramatic development. It is a springtime called the embryonic period that will be followed by a thirty-two week summer, the fetal period, during which the fetus will grow to maturity before birth. By the end of the eighth week, all essential organs and systems are established. Its body acquires a characteristic human shape, if not proportion. The eyes, ears, nose and mouth are visible, though the face remains ten days away from a recognizable human profile and appearance. Like spring come upon a garden, different structures and features bud and flower, each in its own time and place, to brighten the womb with life.

Primordial Buds

By the middle of the third week, the embryo has grown to one-eighth of an inch long. It is slightly pinched in the center with one end clearly larger than the other. The primordia, precursors of organs, begin to appear as distinct groups of cells within the ectoderm, mesoderm and endoderm. Once the mesoderm sandwiches itself between the other layers, cells move through it, along the length of the embryo, and lay a rod. Around this rod, the notochord, the spine eventually forms. Above the notochord, the neural tube forms. Narrow openings left at both ends of the neural tube soon shut and the crest, the larger end, swells to fashion the brain. The neural tube gives rise to the nervous system.

At the same time, chunks of mesoderm called somites form in pairs, starting at the pinched waist, on both sides of the neural tube. More than forty pairs of somites form within two weeks to generate muscle, skin and skeletal tissue, including the spinal vertebrae which they so closely resemble. The heart and blood vessels also arise from the mesoderm. Within two or

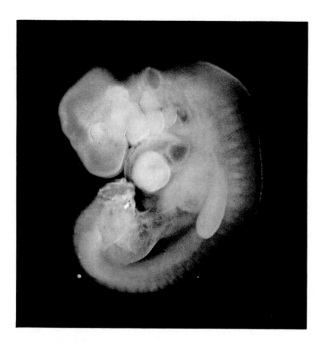

Like a fiery ember, the heart glows within an embryo only four weeks old. Already it pumps blood through lacy blood vessels to the primordia, forerunners of organs. Above the heart and below the head, branchial arches hint of gills, certifying the embryo's share in the common stock of animal life. From head to tail run somites, masses of cells from which the skeleton and muscles grow.

three days, soon after the mesoderm forms, the heart is but two tiny tubes sheathed by muscle cells, which begin to fuse into a single chamber as the third week ends. As the fourth week begins, this crude heart bulges beneath the front of the embryo, like an Adam's apple, and begins to pump blood through simple arteries and veins. This rudimentary circulatory system reaches out to the primordia — esophagus, stomach, liver, pancreas and intestine — all emerging from the endoderm in the belly of the embryo.

Nothing so puzzles embryologists as the way in which cells outfit themselves and trek about to settle different regions of the embryo. Recent experiments with animal embryos have yielded important clues to the fashioning of life. Some cells, like pioneers, make for open frontiers when their home towns get too crowded. Among them are cells which blaze trails by loosing hyaluronic acid, a chemical that clears obstacles and lays paths for other cells to follow. Less sure of how migrating cells choose where to alight, scientists know only that as the concentration of hyaluronic acid around them falls, the cells draw together to found particular tissues and organs.

Where cells settle down, not where they come from, shapes their character. In experiments, cells were taken from the part of the neural tube generating nerves that govern digestion. These were transplanted into another part of the tube that generates nerves responsible for the dilation of the eyes' pupils. The transplanted cells became reflex nerves, the kind that would govern pupil dilation. Like an Easterner gone West, they took on an identity and occupation suited to their new location. Further experiments have confirmed the importance of environment in the development of cells. At the University of Oregon, embryologist James Weston demonstrated that, on their travels, cells meet molecules which show them the ropes, much as an old hand might school a greenhorn. He found that cells from the neural tube, grown in neutral surroundings, became simple pigment cells. But, grown in fibronectin, a chemical common in embryos, identical cells from the neural tube grew into reflex nerves. Weston concluded that cells develop in response to the environment they encounter.

Cells not only adapt to their surroundings but seem to learn from one another. Once they stake a claim, they announce it to neighbors and newcomers alike, proclaiming what part they will take in the community. Testing this idea, scientists removed cells from the belly of a toad embryo and grafted them onto the head of a newt embryo. Told by the newt of their whereabouts, the trespassers adapted themselves as best they could to function as a newt's specialized head cells. Scientists believe similar but more subtle "conversations" between cells normally occur. In the hand, researchers speculate, this process may determine which cells become specific fingers and which, the thumb.

These findings suggest that the environment in which cells move, settle and grow, as well as the relations between them, affects the behavior of genes. Accustomed to casting genes in the leading role of the developmental drama, scientists now suspect that environmental conditions and intercellular signals may script dialogue and stage directions for genes. Just how genes receive and interpret these messages is the outstanding mystery of embryology.

During the second month, the primordia bloom into tissues and organs. From the ectoderm come the tisues and organs with which a child will reach out to the world beyond itself — the tissues of the five senses and the central and peripheral nervous systems. The mesoderm produces tissues that shape and join the body — bone, cartilage and muscle — and vital organs like the heart, liver, kidneys and spleen. From the mesoderm, too, arise blood vessels connecting these organs. The endoderm gives rise to the linings of the digestive, excretory and respiratory tracts as well as several glands.

By the close of the fourth week, the swelling head bows deeply to rest on the heart bulging beneath it. Arms and then legs appear, first as buds. The buds grow into flipperlike plates streaked with rays — faint forerunners of fingers and toes — late in the fifth week. During the next two weeks, hands reach out, drawing forearms, upper arms and shoulders behind them. Legs develop in the same way, but several days behind the pace set by the arms. Halfway

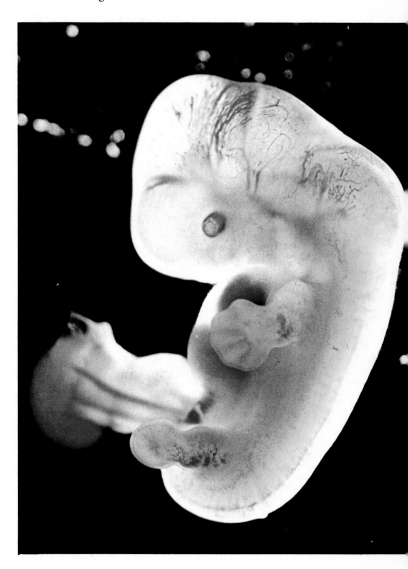

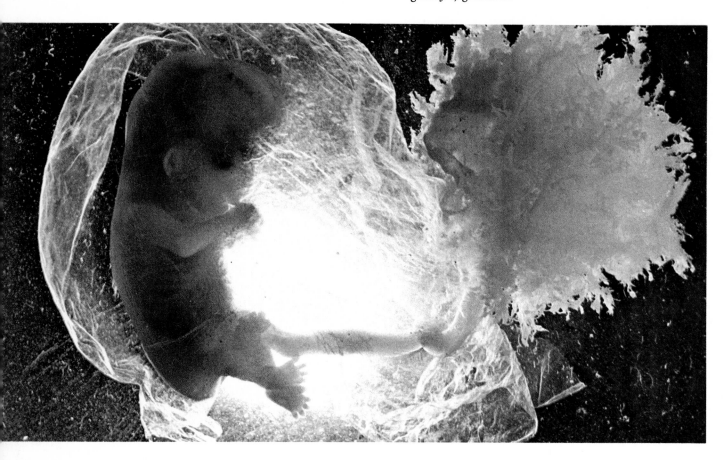

through the sixth week, arms bend at the elbow and, the following week, legs at the knee. Both arms and legs are clasped across the body, fingers and toes nearly touching, in a posture suggesting a yoga position.

The growth of the head outstrips the growth of the trunk. As its sixth week opens, the embryo measures roughly half an inch, half of which is head — a share that holds constant until the eighth week. The face is steadily sculpted. Eyes, ears and nose first appear as pits during the fourth week and the mouth as a crease, a week later. Soon, eyes stand out as black circles while below them darkened shadows hint of ears to come. Nose and mouth evolve like caverns carved by wind and water. The walls of the mouth cavity rise and join, peaking to a vaulted roof, the palate, while above it nostrils open like chimneys. Dominated by an ample crown, facial features change, passing from demonic to inno-

cent in a fleeting fortnight. By the tenth week, the ears have formed, the chin is chiseled and the neck has narrowed. Humanity now covers the embryo's countenance.

As the embryo acquires its human shape and visage, the already beating, single-chambered heart becomes a house of several rooms. By the sixth week, it is pumping blood through an ever-growing labyrinth of vessels. Likewise, the brain divides into its various parts that will house knowledge, store memories, display emotions and control reflexes. From the mesoderm's somites, cartilage and muscle spread to buttress and shape the growing body. Throughout the embryo, save for the skull, cartilage knits an entire skeleton before turning to bone during the sixth week. The respiratory system grows like a grapevine as the windpipe shoots downward. Lungs ripen into clusters entwined with tendrils of breathing passages. The digestive tract develops

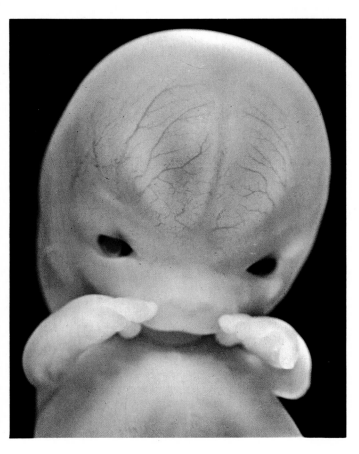

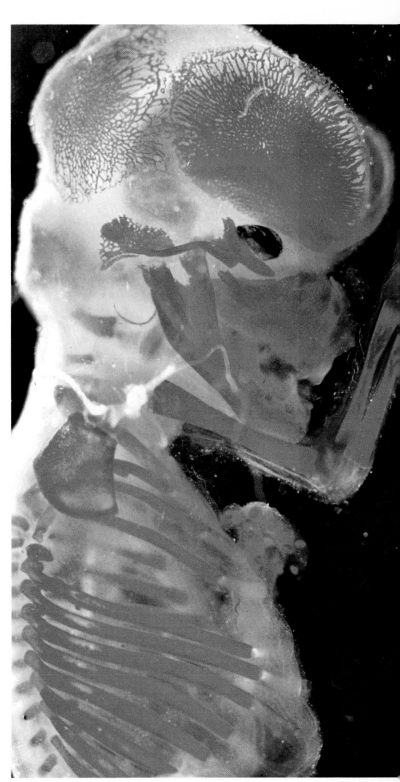

At once vaguely alien yet surely human, the embryo above, of five or six weeks, stares fixedly and reaches squarely toward a future it cannot see in a world it cannot touch. At seven weeks, the skeleton of the embryo, right, begins to turn from cartilage to bone, its metamorphosis betrayed to the camera by stain. In time, membranes will layer one atop another, making the skull to shield the developing brain.

quickly along with the stomach, which produces its first digestive juices in the second trimester, about the twentieth week. Soon afterward the liver and kidneys start performing simple tasks.

As it develops, the embryo assumes shapes and sports features reminiscent of other forms of animal life. Once it was thought that the human embryo climbed each branch of the evolutionary animal tree — fish, amphibian, reptile and mammal — before reaching mankind at the top. Five branchial arches, wrinkling below the head during the fourth and fifth weeks, looked like gills. Similarly the tail, which steadily recedes between the fourth and seventh weeks, hinted at a likeness to many other species.

During its early development the embryo relies on makeshift sources of nourishment while the placenta matures, a process completed in four months. From the beginning, the placenta develops through the cooperative efforts of mother and child and, when complete, consists of parts fashioned by each. On the heels of implantation, circulation begins. Where the trophoblast has implanted itself, the endometrium has eroded. Villi, sprouted from the trophoblast, enlarge and spread, choking the pools of maternal blood like water hyacinths. They join to form larger blood vessels running through the umbilical cord, woven from the body stalk and fetal membranes. The amniotic cavity expands. Its membrane fuses with the chorion to enclose the body stalk, together with its blood vessels. Like an underground cable, the umbilical cord carries two arteries that remove deoxygenated blood from the embryo, and a vein bringing oxygen-rich blood. Meanwhile, arteries and veins in the mother's womb, shaped like corkscrews, spill blood into the endometrium's pools. As the two networks of blood vessels spread, one from child and the other from mother, the placenta grows.

Occupying a third of the uterus, the placenta is a flattened, round disk about seven inches wide, an inch thick and weighing a pound. Its maternal side is divided into lobes, sectioned by the villi running through it. Membranes covering the fetal side lend it a smooth, glassy look, lined with arteries and veins radiating from the umbilical cord near its center.

Though temporary, the placenta is a remarkable organ. Bringing oxygen and taking carbon dioxide from the fetal blood stream, it serves as a lung. It also nourishes the fetus, providing water, minerals, proteins, vitamins, carbohydrates and fats. Most of these substances pass through the placenta from the mother's blood, but others, especially proteins, are manufactured by the placenta. No other organ, not even the liver, produces protein at the same pace. Acting as a kidney, the placenta removes the waste products of fetal metabolism. Primarily a conduit for nutrients and wastes, the placenta is also a barrier, blocking the passage of many substances potentially dangerous to the fetus, including bacteria and drugs. Finally, the placenta replaces the work of the corpus luteum as the mother's hormone factory, producing progesterone, estrogen and other hormones required by pregnancy.

From Embryo to Fetus

From the eighth week onward, when an embryo becomes a fetus, sheer growth overshadows manifold development. Only the face and the external genitalia remain to mature in the first weeks of the fetal period. Just as grain sprouted in springtime ripens to fullness over summer, so does the fetus's weight increase during the last thirty-two weeks of pregnancy. In an average fetus, weight multiplies six hundred times, rising from less than an ounce to seven pounds. In this time, too, the fetus grows to its full length of twenty inches. With growth, proportions change. Fetal limbs and trunk grow while the head shrinks from half to only a fourth of its stature.

Finishing touches are added to appearance, around the twentieth week when hair, eyebrows and eyelashes lend definition to the face and head. Fingernails and toenails complete the delicate limbs. Fine downy hair, called lanugo, covers the limbs and trunk, only to disappear by birth. Growing faster than the tissue beneath it, the skin wrinkles, foreshadowing the look of old age. Not until the last two months will the wizened body change when the fetus puts on weight and its countenance grows young.

Not only does the fetus look more and more like a child, it also begins to behave like one.

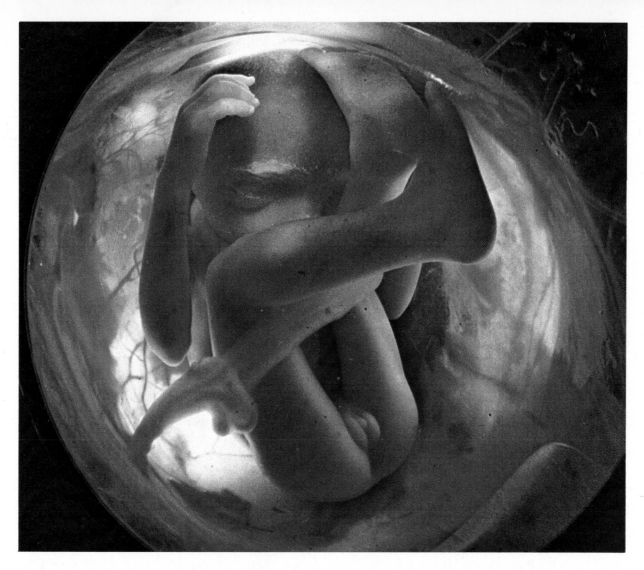

After just eight weeks, the fetus, unknown to its mother, flexes its body and nods its head. In another six weeks, it moves its limbs to avoid discomfort. Early in the fourth month, the fetus begins to swallow, soon taking in the amniotic fluid around it and hiccuping from the effort. Thumb sucking, the most characteristic of infant gestures, is mastered a month later. Also from the fifth month, the fetus dozes and wakes, rolling into a favorite position to sleep and limbering up on rising. Feathery flutterings tell the mother of the coming of the quickening, when she first feels her child stir within her. Later, she will wince at sharp thumps as the fetus becomes more boisterous. Marie Antoinette, who followed her husband, King Louis XVI of France, to the guillotine, once petitioned the throne, saying, "I have come, Sire, to complain of one of your subjects who has been so audacious as to kick me in the belly." The fetus acquires the grasping reflex of

the newborn during the sixth month. In the month before birth, when hungry or annoyed, the fetus cries on its mother's unhearing ears.

As the organs developed in the first eight weeks grow, they begin to function like an orchestra tuning and rehearsing. After twenty weeks, fetal heartbeat sounds through a stethoscope. Because the lungs remain collapsed until they draw breath at birth, the fetus's heart pumps blood laden with oxygen from its mother's lungs. Almost two-thirds its adult size, the brain commands a lively nervous system which distinguishes tastes and smells and responds to light and sound.

The fetus needs all the time Nature grants it, thirty-eight to forty-two weeks, before venturing safely into the outside world. If that time is cut short, it must be extended by creating, as nearly as possible, conditions outside the womb to match those inside. When the fetus is twenty-

FROM CONCEPTION TO BIRTH

Birth is the finale of an unbroken chain of events, each with myriad aspects. Less than two weeks after conception, the blastocyst implants itself in the wall of the womb and begins to form both the placenta and the embryo. After eight weeks, the organs and systems essential for life have developed. Over the remaining thirty weeks, the fetal period, these organs and systems grow rapidly and begin functioning. They are sustained by the placenta, which matures by the fourth month. All the while, the fetus steadily acquires a childlike visage and stature.

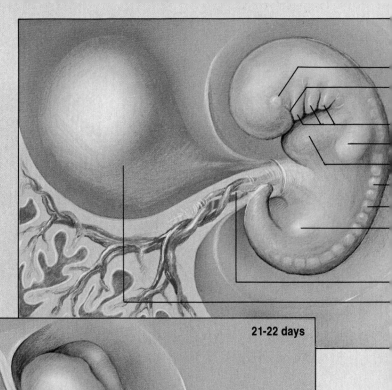

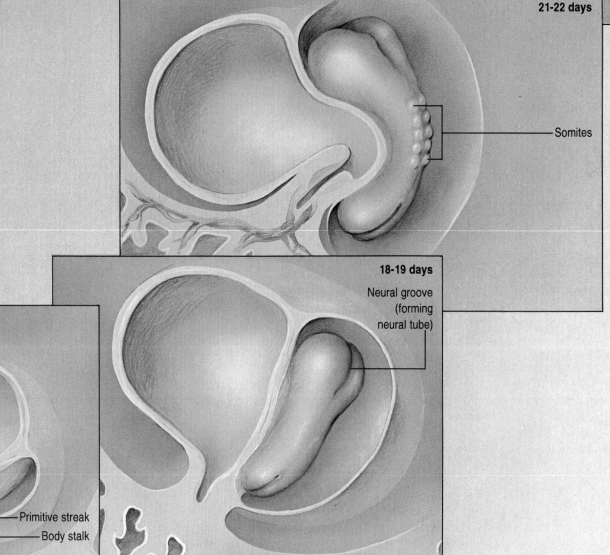

days

tocyst

21-22 days

— Somites

18-19 days

Neural groove
(forming
neural tube)

Primitive streak

Body stalk

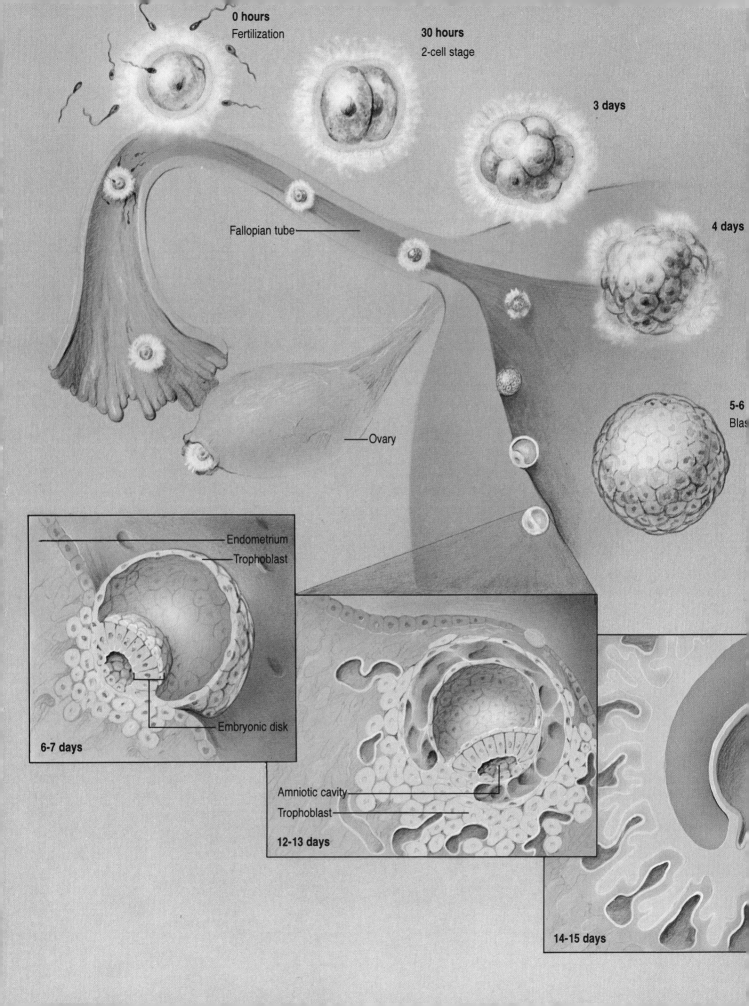

0 hours
Fertilization

30 hours
2-cell stage

3 days

4 days

5-6
Blas

Fallopian tube

Ovary

Endometrium
Trophoblast

Embryonic disk

6-7 days

Amniotic cavity
Trophoblast

12-13 days

14-15 days

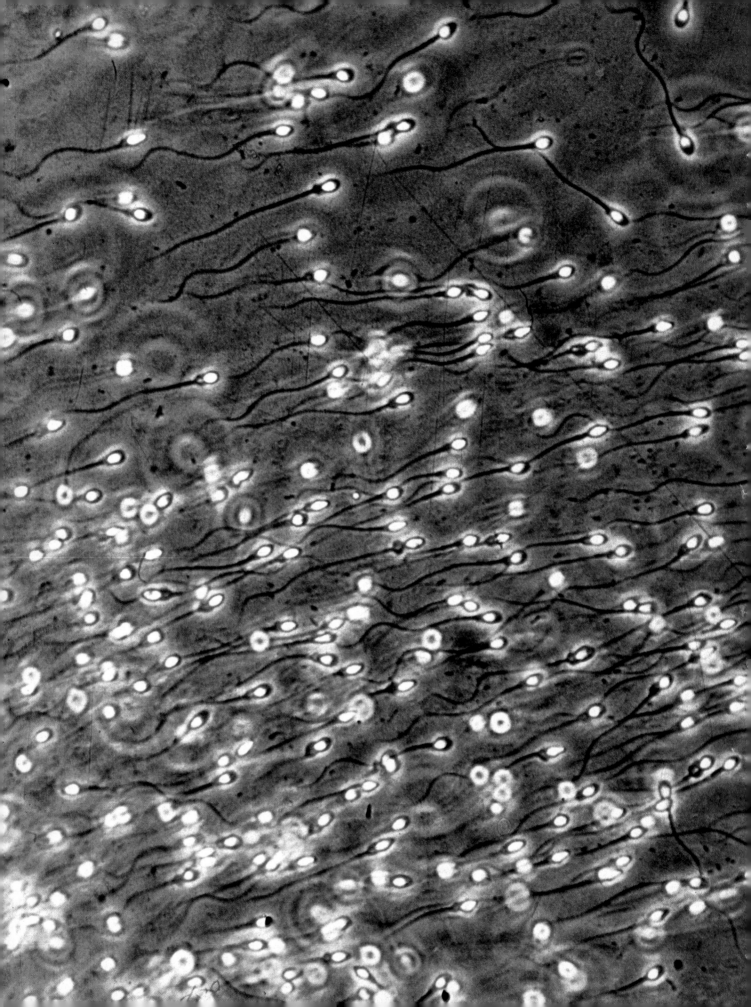

*Until after the Renaissance, a sense
of propriety and lack of cadavers
fostered misunderstanding of female
anatomy. This sixteenth-century
print of a pregnant woman was
taken from a classical drawing.*

*As contour lines plot terrain on a
map, so the camera traces changing
landscapes of pregnancy, right. The
technique of stereophotography is
used widely in Europe to measure
the growth of pregnant women.*

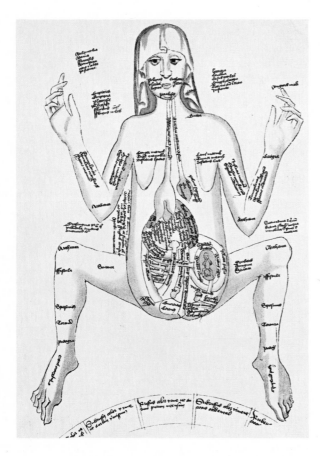

pregnancy. Estrogens prepare the uterus to receive, nourish and house the child. They enlarge
and soften the pubic joints, ligaments and tissues
to ease the child's birth. And they ready the
breasts for the time when the child will suckle.
Progesterone forestalls contractions of the uterus,
which would cause the pregnancy to miscarry,
and complements the work of the estrogens.

Miscarriages occur during the first twenty
weeks of pregnancy from causes still somewhat
obscure. One inquiry revealed that in nearly
two-thirds of the miscarriages studied, the fetus
or its membranes were abnormally developed.
The scientists attributed some of these abnormalities to errant behavior of chromosomes. Other
studies suggest that the uterus's inadequate preparation for implantation, perhaps due to hormone
deficiencies, may be a major cause, particularly in
women who habitually miscarry. Serious infections and diseases, especially bacterial ones, are
also known to cause miscarriage. Falls, so fright-
ening to the mother, rarely end pregnancies. The
fetus is well protected against such accidents.

Essential to pregnancy, hormones have other
effects, some that are inconvenient or uncom-
fortable for the mother. Both estrogens and progesterone slacken smooth muscle, muscle not
consciously controlled, throughout the mother's
body. Relaxed tissue in the urinary and digestive
tracts makes for frequent urination, along with a
greater chance of urinary infection and constipa-
tion. Estrogens affect connective tissue, cartilage
and ligaments, commonly causing backache, especially late in pregnancy when an upright posture is needed to offset the forward weight of the
uterus. By loosening pelvic joints, hormones set
the waddling gait, what Shakespeare called "the
proud walk of pregnancy," of expectant mothers.
Estrogens soften fibrous tissue, scoring the skin
on the abdomen, hips and breasts with stretch
marks. They lessen the output of pepsin, a digestive enzyme, which brings on nausea. They also
prompt the kidneys to retain more water, which
can lead to edema, an excess of fluid in the body,
especially late in pregnancy. Gums softened by
estrogens may bleed from the pressure of a
toothbrush or from chewing food. Together, estrogens and progesterone paint the "mask of

four weeks old, it can survive outside the womb
if it must, but requires special and intensive care
to do so. Both its kidneys and liver begin to function as early as the twelfth week, but the kidneys
do not mature until the thirty-sixth week and the
liver does not perform all its tasks until well after
birth. Above all, the lungs, among the slowest of
the organs to mature, grow until the child is eight
years old. If born premature, the baby cannot
capture the oxygen it needs.

A Mother's Changing Body

To carry, nurture and deliver her child, the mother's body undergoes myriad changes, many of
them caused by the hormones which sustain her
pregnancy. Hormones are produced chiefly by
the placenta, sometimes in partnership with the
two adrenal glands and the liver of the fetus.
Various forms of estrogen, at least twenty-seven,
and progesterone are the principal agents of

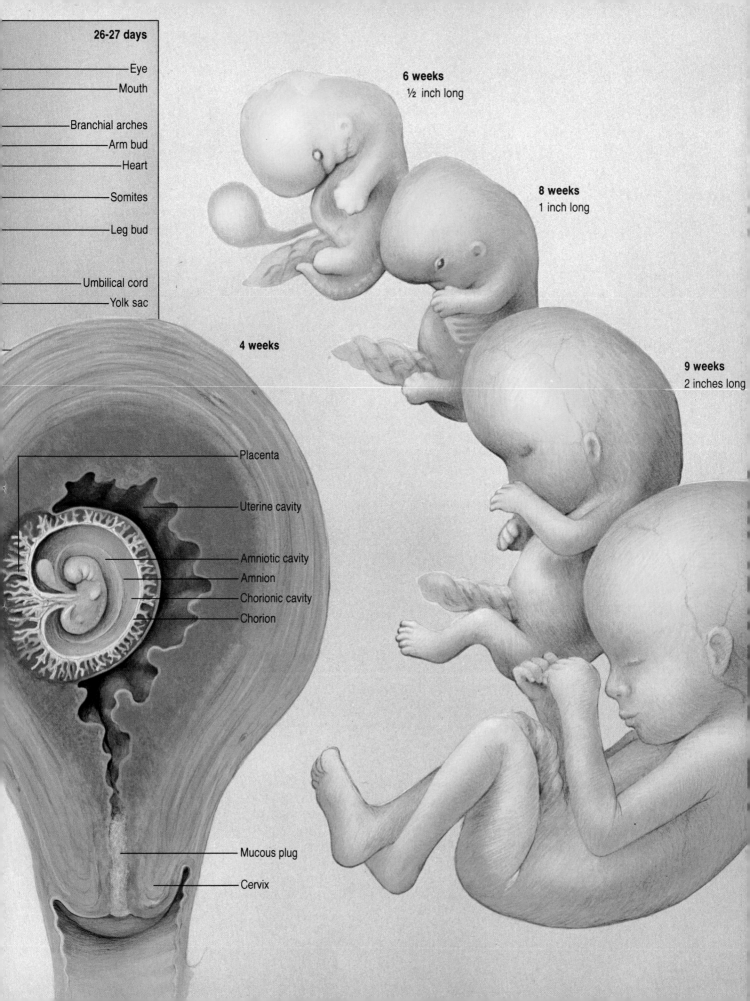

26-27 days

Eye

Mouth

Branchial arches

Arm bud

Heart

Somites

Leg bud

Umbilical cord

Yolk sac

4 weeks

6 weeks
½ inch long

8 weeks
1 inch long

9 weeks
2 inches long

Placenta

Uterine cavity

Amniotic cavity

Amnion

Chorionic cavity

Chorion

Mucous plug

Cervix

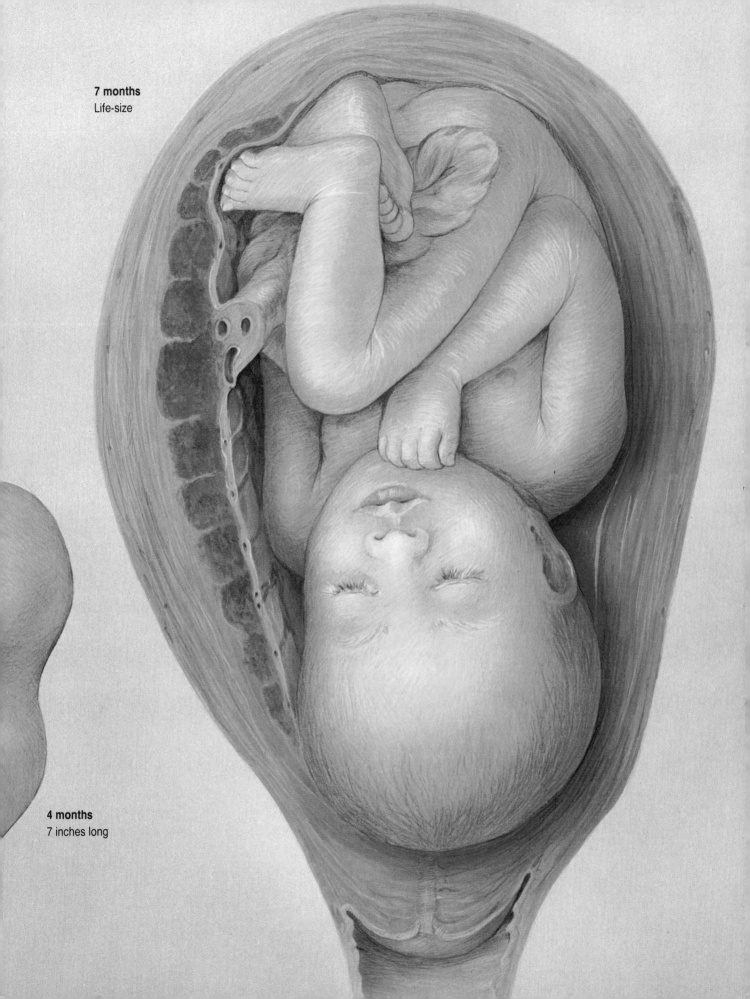

7 months
Life-size

4 months
7 inches long

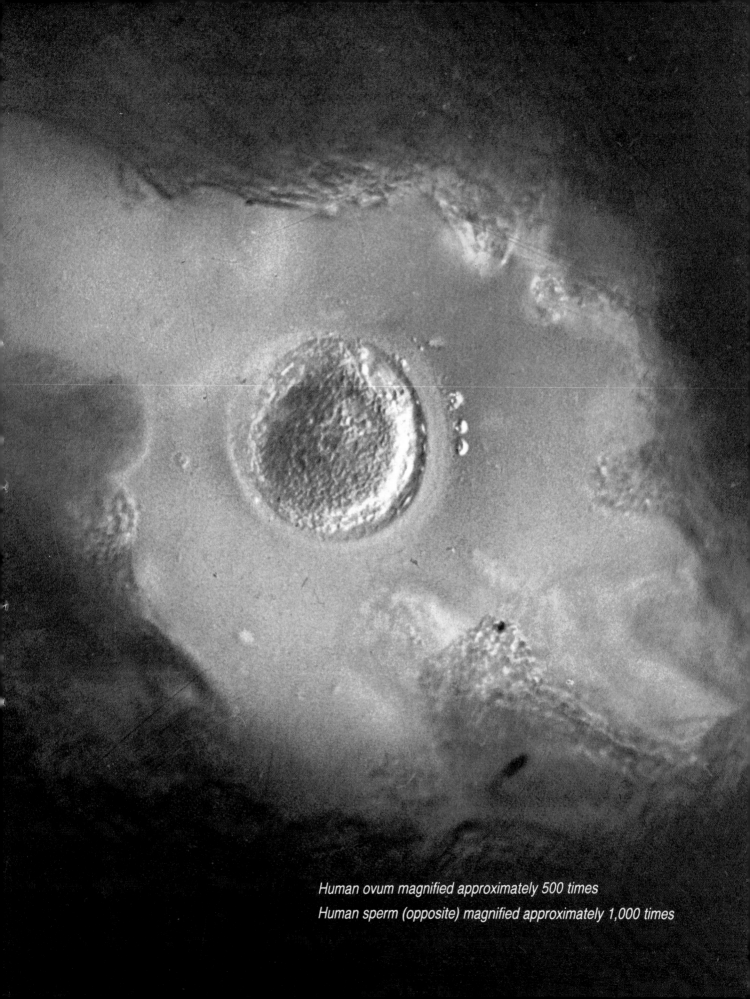

Human ovum magnified approximately 500 times

Human sperm (opposite) magnified approximately 1,000 times

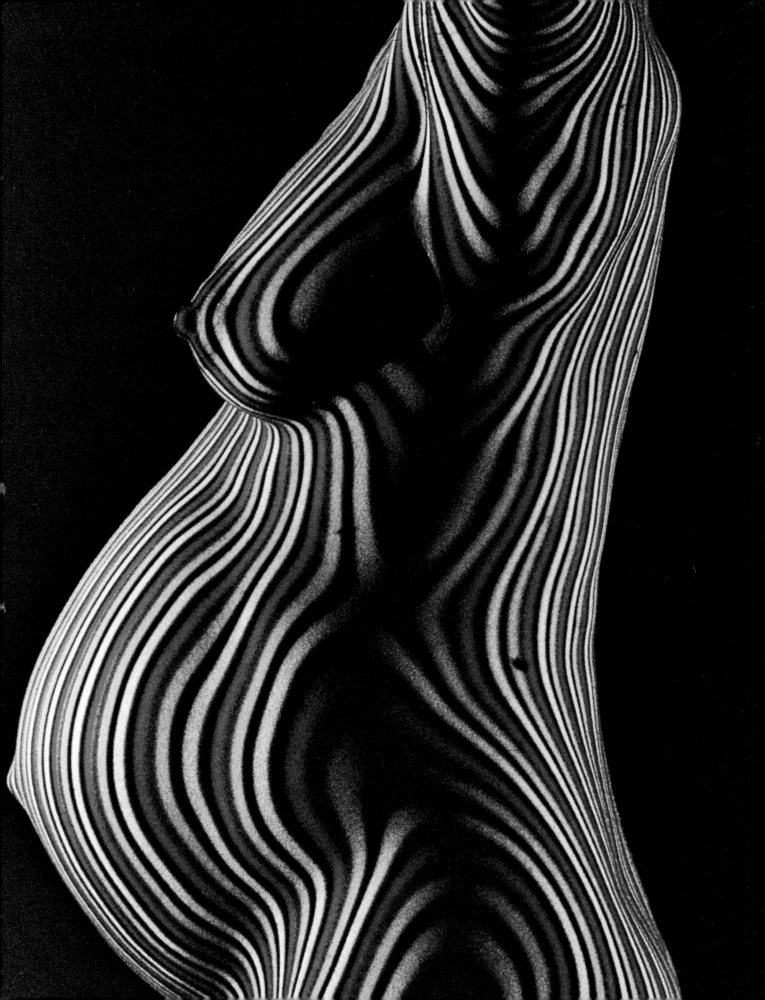

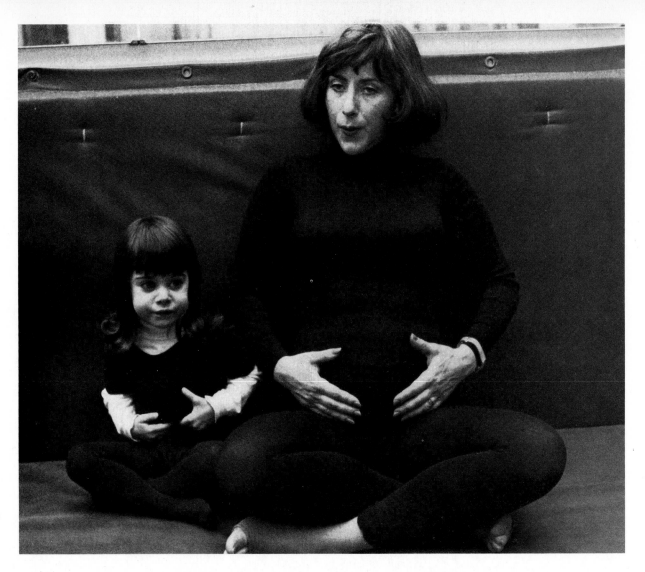

pregnancy," or chloasma, darkening the skin around the nose and cheeks and the nipples.

The hormones have a marked impact on blood circulation. Blood volume rises nearly 50 percent, a safeguard against heavy loss during delivery. Estrogens heighten the tendency of blood to coagulate, increasing the risk of clotting, or thrombosis. Greater blood flow in the pelvic region slows the return of blood to the heart. Sluggish blood flow may cause varicose veins in the legs, hemorrhoids and lightheadedness or fainting.

With proper care and nutrition, none of these conditions need threaten mother or fetus. The expectant mother visits her physician regularly, once a month during the first two trimesters, then every two weeks during the eighth month and, finally, each week during the ninth month. Her first visit may be lengthy. The doctor gives her a complete physical examination and takes a medical history of the patient and her family, in-

quiring particularly about prior pregnancies, chronic illness and hereditary diseases. On subsequent visits, the mother's blood is monitored, especially for any sign of anemia. Her urine is checked for glucose, a possible sign of gestational diabetes. This form of the disease is peculiar to pregnancy and, if untreated, complicates carrying and delivering the child.

Late in pregnancy, the doctor watches for sharp rises in blood pressure and urine protein which may signal preeclampsia-eclampsia, a disorder associated with high blood pressure. It is gravely threatening to mother and fetus. Most common among young women bearing their first child, preeclampsia-eclampsia strikes close to full term. Preeclampsia, the first stage, blurs vision, and causes severe headaches or recurrent dizziness. When spotted and treated, preeclampsia can be checked, forestalling eclampsia itself. Marked by convulsions, eclampsia takes a heavy toll on mothers and children. A patient suffering from preeclampsia is confined to bed, encouraged to rest and sometimes sedated with medication. Some doctors recommend a salt-free diet with plentiful fluids, but other doctors think that some sodium is necessary for mother and fetus.

The physician measures the size of the uterus from visit to visit to ensure that the fetus is growing regularly. And, from the twentieth week, the fetal heartbeat is closely monitored. More and more routine, examination by ultrasound takes a sure measure of the growth and development of the fetus. For the most part, the mother cares for herself. Above all she needs a sound, balanced and regular diet. The doctor tells her what should be eaten and what should be avoided. More protein in her diet is desirable, though the belief that a high-protein diet significantly reduces the risk of complications remains unfounded. Even the most finely balanced diet may need to be supplemented with minerals and vitamins to meet the added demands. Pregnant women often develop aversions to certain foods and cravings for others. Pica, a craving for bizarre substances, can be harmful. Red clay and laundry starch are perennial American favorites that are, not surprisingly, hazardous.

Doctors have treated weight gain as designers have fixed hemlines. Not long ago, they watched the scale very closely, scolding patients who gained too quickly and too much. Today, many doctors are as lenient as their predecessors were strict. But others urge mothers to limit added pounds, believing that too many can trouble the pregnancy and the delivery. Because weight is more easily gained than lost, they say, a mother can fail to regain her figure — often a source of anxiety after childbirth.

Apart from diet, exercise is a necessary part of pregnancy's regimen. Keeping fit eases the strain of pregnancy, readying the body for delivery and hastening the mother's return to form. Expectant mothers can choose from a variety of formal exercise programs and physical activities suited to their condition. There are special exercises designed to enhance breathing technique and muscle tone, aimed specifically to prepare the mother for the rigors of delivery.

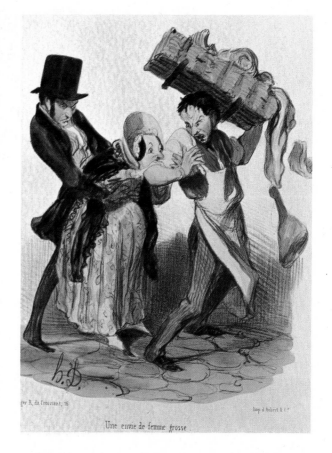

Une envie de femme grosse.

Good health, sustained by diet and exercise, stiffens resistance to infectious disease. Once scourges of pregnancy, the impacts of infectious disease can now be greatly lessened or altogether avoided by an alert and informed mother. Such diseases are carried by tiny organisms, mainly bacteria and viruses. Bacterial diseases usually cause miscarriages and stillbirths. Viral infections generally have a mild effect on the mother, but may seriously damage the developing embryo, especially in early pregnancy. In America, most bacterial diseases have been brought under control. If, against the odds, the expectant mother is stricken with a serious illness like pneumonia, there is a good chance she can be successfully treated with antibiotics. By the time they reach their childbearing years, most women are immune to the most common viral infections — measles, mumps and chicken pox. They probably have also been inoculated against influenza, smallpox and poliomyelitis. Because vaccinations themselves may harm the fetus, immunity must be established before pregnancy.

Hazards and Hard Learned Lessons

Since the seventeenth century, when newborns scarred by smallpox were first observed, science has known that disease can pass from mother to fetus. But infectious disease was not linked to other birth defects until 1941, when Australian doctor N. M. Gregg linked German measles contracted during pregnancy to cataracts veiling babies' eyes. Unlike most common viral infections of childhood, German measles, or rubella, does not always confer immunity and can return to strike a pregnant woman. This discovery led Gregg to suspect all viral infections which, thanks to subsequent research, today stand convicted of causing a wide range of birth defects. Outbreaks of German measles in the United States in 1964 and 1970 revealed its severe impact. During the first month of pregnancy, the most critical period, the embryo of a mother taken with rubella runs a 50 percent risk of being deformed. Over the next three months, the risk lessens to about 30 percent. A fetus's eyes, ears, heart and brain may be impaired. The odds in favor of such defects and the anxiety they cause the mother lead many physicians to recommend abortion after exposure to German measles.

Venereal diseases are particularly insidious during pregnancy, especially because their symptoms are seldom apparent to the mother. Syphilis has been detected in fetuses as early as the eighth week of pregnancy and unless diagnosed and treated before the sixteenth week, it will harm the fetus. If it does, it often causes deformity or death. If left untreated, gonorrhea also has devastating effects on the fetus, most often leaving the eyes inflamed and the joints arthritic. Venereal diseases, like most others, can be contained by swift diagnosis and treatment.

Recent research has revealed further hazards for mother and child from cigarettes, alcohol and drugs. Cigarette smoking, so harmful to health, poses particular perils during pregnancy. Those mothers who smoke run a significant risk of miscarriage, 30 to 70 percent higher than pregnant women who do not smoke. The risk rises with the number of cigarettes smoked. Fetal deaths after eighteen weeks rise sharply among smoking mothers. Premature delivery is more common among mothers who smoke than among those who do not. Smoking, according to a 1981 report by the Surgeon General, accounts for 13 percent of premature births in the United States.

Evidence from other countries suggests that children of smokers suffer, too. Some studies indicate that infants of smoking mothers have a mortality rate anywhere from 10 to 100 percent higher than children of nonsmokers. The rate varies with other factors, such as class origins and prenatal history, which also may place the child at risk. Finnish findings, paralleled elsewhere, show that children of smoking mothers fall ill more often, particularly with respiratory complaints. They also seem more susceptible to sudden infant death syndrome (SIDS).

Alcohol, like tobacco, endangers the future of the fetus. The alarm against alcohol is an ancient one. In the city-states of Sparta and Carthage newly-weds were forbidden drink. Aristotle scorned "foolish, drunken or hare-brained women" who "bring forth children like unto themselves, morose and languid." In the Roman Republic, women were likewise not allowed alcohol. Similar prohibitions were upheld by folk tradition for centuries. Between 1720 and 1750, cheap gin flooded Britain, touching off the "Gin Epidemic." Children, one report noted, were "born weak and sickly, and often look shrivel'd and old." Like observations persisted, but not until drinking patterns changed markedly after the Second World War, when women began to drink more, did the impact of alcohol on the unborn attract intense scientific attention.

Undertaken in France in 1968, the first modern study reported low birth weights and misshapen facial bones together with signs of mental and emotional abnormalities in the children of heavy drinkers. Led by Kenneth Jones, a team from the University of Washington School of Medicine in Seattle confirmed the French findings by the early 1970s, dubbing the condition fetal alcohol syndrome, or FAS. Subsequent inquiries have described the syndrome more fully.

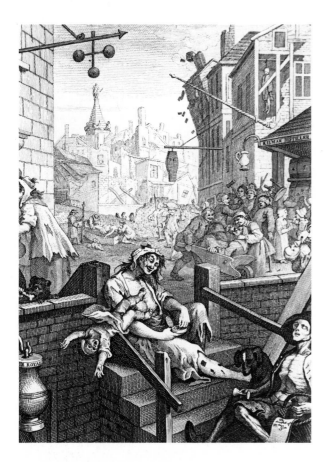

Brimming with telling vignettes of depravity, debauchery and death, William Hogarth's engraving Gin Lane *sternly indicted the wave of gin-drinking that washed over early eighteenth-century England. Fast earning the epithet "Mother's Ruin," gin, what Hogarth called the "Damn'd Cup," also affected children. Contemporary observers commented on the blighted faces, stunted physiques and dull minds of babies born to heavy drinkers.*

Evidence indicates that a mother's heavy drinking may lead to many physical and mental shortcomings in her child. Parts of the brain may fail to develop properly or even to develop at all. Eyes may not mature. Cleft palates and deformed limbs appear among children of heavy drinkers. Some children have abnormally developed hearts or genitalia. Nor are mental retardation and deficiency uncommon. The dangers of light drinking, defined as one ounce or less, have not been demonstrated. Alcohol consumption falls spontaneously and significantly after conception, even among heavy drinkers, perhaps because of the nausea accompanying pregnancy. Few doctors demand total abstinence, but all remind their patients that a pregnant woman never drinks alone.

Recent tragedies have highlighted the dangers of drugs, dangers all the more sinister because the drugs were prescribed with confidence by physicians. In the autumn of 1960, pediatricians throughout West Germany were bewildered to find grotesquely deformed infants brought to their clinics in significant numbers. Hands grew almost directly from shoulders and legs, though longer, were shortened and twisted. Many suffered from malformations of the ear, digestive tract, heart and circulatory system. Almost all bore a strawberry mark, running from the forehead to the upper lip, as if they needed this harmless sign to mark their wretched plight. Mercifully, neither their intellect nor personality was marred. Most pediatricians had never seen such deformities, certainly not in an individual child. The deformed limbs suggested phocomelia — from the Greek *phoke,* for "seal," and *melos,* meaning "limb" — a disorder so rare that few physicians witnessed it in a lifetime. During the next year, few West German pediatricians had not seen children with phocomelia, usually accompanied by internal deformities.

In November 1961, a Hamburg pediatrician, Widukind Lenz, disclosed that he had tentatively traced the tragedy to a new and very popular sedative called thalidomide. Lenz's hunch, confirmed by further research, was sound. Taken between the third and eighth weeks, sometimes by women ignorant of their pregnancy, thalidomide disrupted the normal course of embryonic development. Almost at once, drugs containing thalidomide were taken off the market in West Germany and soon afterward they were banned around the world. But for 10,000 children in a score of countries, the ban came too late. Thanks to Frances Oldham Kelsey, medical officer of the Food and Drug Administration, who stubbornly resisted the blandishments of the William S. Merrell Company, which sought to market the drug in the United States, thalidomide never reached American pharmacies.

Not all drugs strike with the sudden fury of thalidomide. Some, like ghosts, haunt the body long after they first enter it. In 1966, a fifteen-year-old girl saw Arthur Herbst of Massachusetts General Hospital. She complained of continual vaginal bleeding. At first stymied, Herbst finally diagnosed a rare form of cancer known as clear-cell adenocarcinoma. Within four years, Herbst treated seven cases, more than the total number reported in all the world's medical literature. He found that the mothers of his patients, all young women, had taken diethylstilbestrol (DES), during their pregnancies.

During the 1940s, George Van Siclen Smith, head of the department of gynecology at Harvard Medical School, and his wife, biochemist Olive Watkins Smith, began championing DES, a synthetic estrogen. They claimed that DES encouraged implantation and prevented miscarriage in patients with troubled histories and, curiously, that it could "make a normal pregnancy more normal." In St. Louis, Willard Allen was puzzled. His work with rabbits indicated that supplemental estrogen was "very deleterious to the fetus" and could "prevent implantation and produce abortion." Soon, studies conducted in Chicago and New Orleans concluded that DES had "no therapeutic value in pregnancy" and might have caused fetal deaths and premature births. Despite such suspicions, between the 1940s and the early 1970s, millions of pregnant women were given DES, often unknowingly.

By the late 1960s, evidence mounted that DES was, as Herbst suspected, responsible for abnormalities in the genital tract of young women beginning to be called "DES daughters." Further research has shown that in most cases the abnormalities are benign, though potentially cancerous. Abnormalities appear, usually between the ages of eighteen and twenty-three, then recede. The daughters whose own births were allegedly eased by DES have difficulty bearing children of their own. Although most can have children, some suffer repeated miscarriages, ectopic pregnancies and premature deliveries. Since the male genitalia form during the seventh week of development, before DES was generally taken, DES daughters outnumber their "brothers." But sons also experience genital-tract problems, and may have an increased risk of sterility and cancer.

The use of DES during pregnancy was finally restricted by the Food and Drug Administration in 1971. But it is still used to suppress lactation in mothers not wishing to breast-feed their babies, to ease menopause and to treat women who have lost their ovaries or who suffer breast cancer. Paradoxically, it is an ingredient of the so-called morning-after contraceptive pill, thwarting pregnancies it was originally intended to enhance. The thalidomide and DES fiascos sparked legal proceedings and sharp political debate from which more responsible testing, marketing and prescribing of drugs emerged. Both were hard learned lessons on the dangers of taking drugs during the early weeks of pregnancy.

Biologically and psychologically, pregnancy is a powerful experience testing character as well as body. Hopes and fears of pregnancy are constant companions of sexually active women and, when it happens, their response may range from delight to deep despair. Initial dismay is a common reaction. It implies no rejection of the child, for women seem at first to separate pregnancy from parenthood. By the fifth month, when the fetus has quickened, the mother has identified it as an individual. She may give her child a pet name, anticipate its gender, even foresee its career. Stroking her swollen belly, she offers caresses which are returned by movements in response to her touch. As birth nears, the physical strains of pregnancy return to slow her movement, tire her body and disturb her rest. Readying a home for her newborn, the mother looks with mounting impatience toward giving birth — "I want to be over and done with it!"

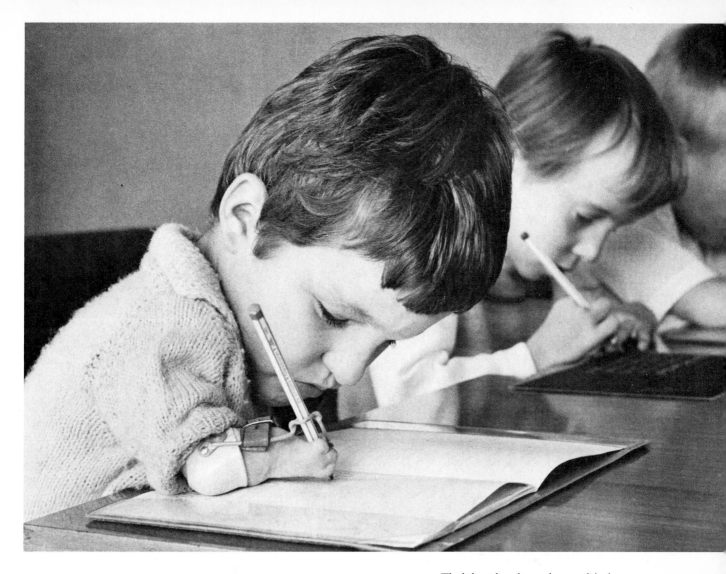

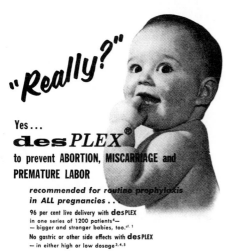

Thalidomide, above, damaged bodies but spared minds. Klaus, his limbs stunted and twisted by thalidomide, works at mastering writing in his West German kindergarten. Devices like Klaus's enabled thalidomide children, now in their twenties, to use their bodies to express their minds. Confidently prescribed to a generation of expectant mothers, diethylstilbestrol (DES), left, has since haunted their teen-age children with fears of genital cancer and reproductive problems.

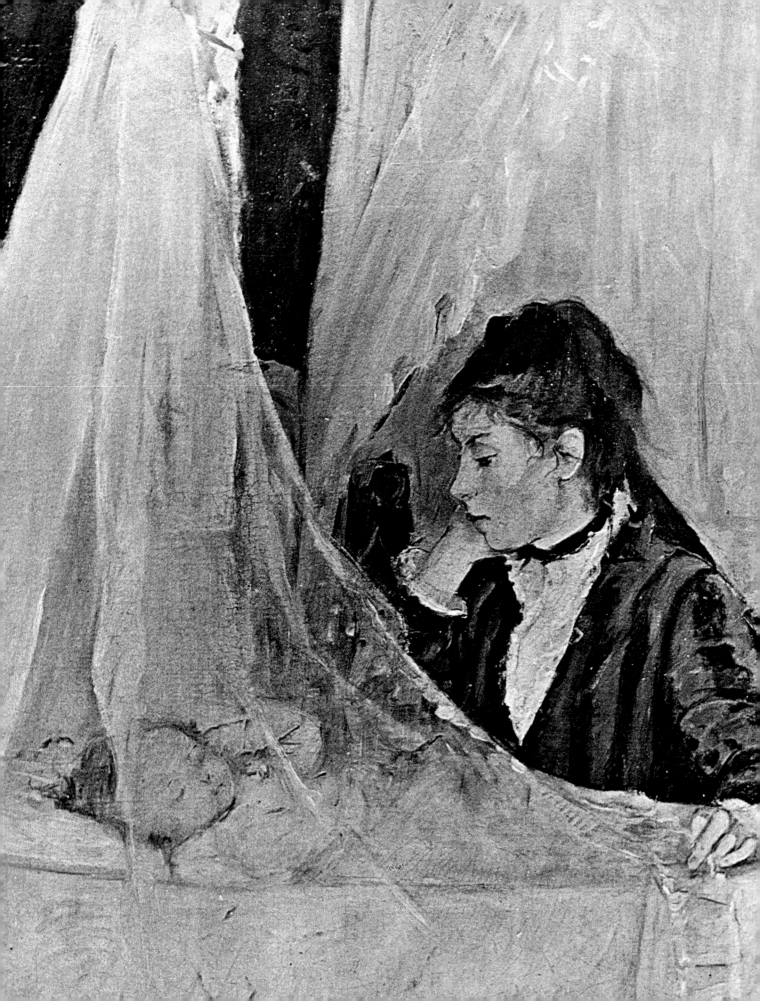

Chapter 4

Of Woman Born

Childbirth transcends biology. Fears, myths and priorities are as much a part of birth as are contractions, pain and a baby's cries. The physical process itself differs little from one birth to the next. Yet, as a social event, childbirth is unique, an expression of its time and culture. We shape it as an artist shapes clay.

A small and squat statue sculpted by a Colima Indian 1,500 years ago in what is now Mexico, shows a woman in labor, her face taut with concentration, her hands pressed on her distended belly. Not long ago, the terra cotta figurine made its way to Denmark, included in an exhibition of pre-Columbian art. For the duration of the show the woman endured her endless labor on her back, with her knees drawn up to her body. The position that seemed proper to the Danes was not intended by the Colima artist. He had crafted the laboring woman upright, squatting on her knees.

In many societies, squatting is the traditional posture of birth. Indeed, the horizontal position we know so well is a rarity outside modern society. Mansi women of Siberia, wearing dresses made especially for the birth, hold themselves upright by propping a horizontal bar under their arms during labor. In the American Southwest, women of the Jicarilla Apaches kneel to give birth and clench a vertical stake for support. A Caticugan woman of the Philippines gives birth sitting on a woven mat, with her back propped by pillows stacked against a wall. She braces her feet against wooden blocks when labor pains become severe. A rope suspended from the ceiling gives her something to clutch.

For the Ainu women of northern Japan, the willow tree provides comfort at birth. According to myth, the backbone of the first man came from a willow. The Ainu say that the graceful trees hold the life force of the body. When a woman is pregnant, her family makes offerings of carved willow branches to the goddess of fire

The theme of mother and child, a favorite of artists, reflects time and place, yet is drawn from universal emotions. Childbirth is a blend of biology and ritual, a commonplace event that maintains the mystique of a miracle and holds entranced the pensive mother of Berthe Morisot's 1872 painting, The Cradle.

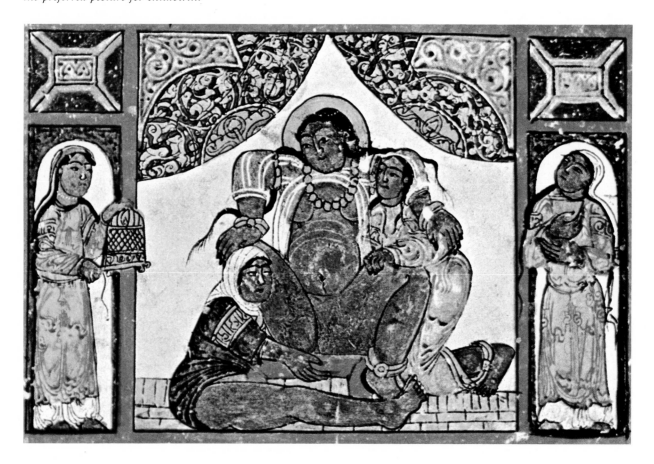

to ensure her good health. If labor grows difficult, the offerings change to pleas. The woman's assistants, female friends and relatives, bounce her up and down on her feet and press on her abdomen to hasten the delivery. As a last resort, they make a desperate request of the goddess:

> From inside myself
> and inside the womb
> there should be a baby
> Gently and easily
> Fire Goddess
> should receive
> and hold it
> safely

Myth weaves inseparably, too, through the lives of Australian aborigines, who give birth as they believe their mythical ancestors did in creating the first human beings. Their *Djanggawul*, or spiritual ancestors, were two sisters who came from across the sea, following the path of the rising sun — a symbol of life. The sisters brought ritual items with them, including a plaited mat that represented the uterus. Aborigine women sleep under such mats and shield themselves from the rituals of the men, which they are forbidden to witness. Male babies are placed on coarse grass after birth, but a female baby is sheltered in the woven mat, confirming the sacredness of the sisters who populated their world.

Across the world and throughout time, childbirth has been, almost exclusively, the domain of women. The role of the midwife — a word deriving from the Middle English "with-woman" — has also been predominately a feminine one. For innumerable centuries, men present at a birth have had limited roles. Husbands could comfort their wives. Religious men and, later, physicians attended only when complications arose.

In Western civilizations, the practice of childbirth has shifted as restlessly as a woman in la-

92

bor. From biblical times until well into the seventeenth century, women usually delivered their babies in a birthing chair, a chair with a horseshoe-shaped seat. In the Middle Ages, birth was a hazardous event for both mother and baby. The laboring woman endured a host of cruelties. To bring on labor, midwives held pepper under her nose to make her sneeze or they made her run up and down stairs. If she had difficulties in labor, her attendants would tie her to a couch, turn it on end and then pound it on the floor. Or they would grab her arms and legs and drop her on the bed again and again. With the high infant mortality rate of the time, saving the infant's soul gained priority over saving its life. A baptismal syringe with a slender, curved tip was designed to anoint the fetus with holy water while it was still in the womb. When the fetus died in the womb or could not be naturally delivered, it was carved out, piece by piece with a sharp, curved hook called a crotchet. This practice was known as "child breaking."

By the sixteenth century, women still dominated midwifery. In 1522, a male physician from Hamburg disguised himself as a midwife to witness a birth. Apparently his costume failed, for he was burned at the stake in punishment. When midwifery finally emerged from the gloom of the Dark Ages, the art took a healthy step forward. In the late sixteenth century, a school for midwives opened in Paris. Textbooks appeared, describing and advising midwifery.

The seventeenth century brought changes to childbirth that had an awesome effect on its future practice. In 1664, French King Louis XIV asked his court physician to tend the labor of his mistress, Louise de La Vallière, who had been forced to hide her pregnancy under layers of clothing. The king feared midwives would reveal her secret. He insisted on watching the birth, so the doctor arranged the patient on a bed rather than a birthing chair, giving Louis a clear view of the proceedings. These two changes, a male physician and a bed instead of a birthing chair, were introduced by little more than a whim of the Sun King. Both practices, however, were established with a device invented by the Chamberlens, an enterprising sixteenth-century English family.

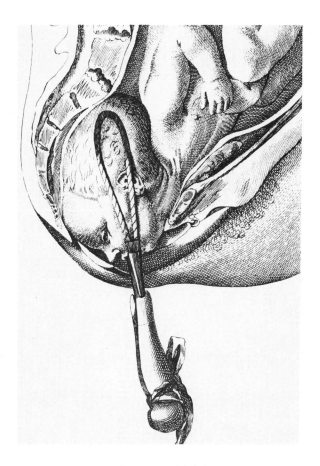

Forceps enabled doctors to overcome difficulties of delivery that once doomed mother and baby alike. These, from an eighteenth-century print, are laced with leather to soften their grip on the baby's head.

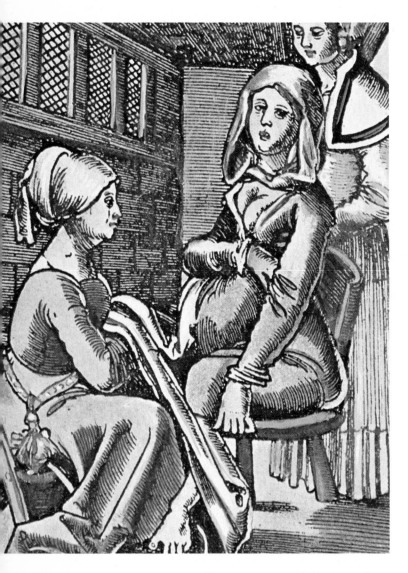

European women of the sixteenth century labored on a birthing stool, fully dressed, in defense of their modesty. This woodcut illustrated one of the earliest manuals written for midwives, published in 1513.

The Chamberlens invented obstetrical forceps. Peter the Elder and his younger brother — also named Peter — were male midwives. With the forceps, the brothers could pull a fetus from the womb without killing it and spare the mother a sometimes long, painful labor. Their impressive success earned them a fortune, which they were determined to increase by keeping their creation a secret. They would blindfold patients before carrying the forceps into the delivery room in an ornate, gilded box.

The son of Peter the Younger, also Peter by name — much to the confusion of historians if not the family — became an obstetrician and perpetuated the family secret. His son, Hugh, also an obstetrician, brought the family's 100-year-old monopoly to an end. Boasting of his skills in the delivery room, he boldly took on the difficult delivery of a dwarfed woman with a deformed pelvis. The effort was disastrous. The woman died, quelling Hugh's confidence and damaging his career. To ease financial difficulties, he sold the forceps to a prominent Dutch male midwife, Roger van Roonhuyse, in 1699.

By the mid-eighteenth century, the use of forceps in birth made the delivery room a place for physicians and lessened the role of the midwife. The birthing chair, too, lost favor. Doctors could manipulate the forceps far more easily when the patient reclined on a bed.

The Forces of Birth

A variety of childbirth practices have followed cycles of favor and disfavor. Today, the midwife and the birthing chair have been reintroduced. Despite the external changes time and culture have brought to the event of birth, the body prepares for it in a cycle that remains untouched by season or style. The uterus primes itself with gentle, periodic contractions throughout pregnancy. In the ninth month, just like an athlete in training, the uterus begins to flex its muscle in earnest when the contractions gradually increase in frequency, culminating in the aptly named process called labor.

Labor is the means by which the uterus expels the fetus and the placenta, the afterbirth that has ceased to be useful. Some physicians believe that

*Reintroduced and modernized, the
birthing stool is gaining popularity
today. Made of fiber glass, the
birthing chair may dramatically
shorten the stages of a woman's
labor, hastening the baby's delivery.*

labor starts once the uterus becomes fully extended. Premature labor occurs frequently in multiple pregnancies, possibly because the uterus reaches full extension sooner when the mother is carrying more than one baby. But this theory does not account for the variety of complications in labor. The body may go into labor to cast out a dead fetus before the uterus reaches full extension. A decrease in the concentration of the hormone progesterone, which inhibits contractions, may also be a mechanism. Progesterone is concentrated where the placenta joins the uterus, ensuring that regular uterine contractions do not jar it loose. As the fetus grows, the rest of the uterus proportionately increases until it presumably overrules progesterone's influence, permitting increased uterine activity.

Other body chemicals may also have a role in the onset of labor. Oxytocin, a hormone secreted by the posterior lobe of the pituitary gland, the body's "master gland" nestled beneath the brain, is known to be a uterine stimulant. Synthetic forms of this hormone are used to induce labor or increase the strength of contraction. The uterus becomes more receptive to oxytocin as pregnancy nears its conclusion, but researchers have not found evidence of an increase in its production. Labor in humans and other animals can also occur in a normal fashion without the hormonal influence of the posterior pituitary. Certain prostaglandins, fatty acids, help prepare the cervix for dilation. Scientists know these substances are also able to cause uterine contractions any time during pregnancy and believe they play a major role in bringing on labor. A group of compounds called catecholamines has a similar function, but it is not clear how they contribute to labor.

More recent work suggests that the fetus itself may have something to do with the onset of labor. This modern idea appears to have a superficial counterpart in the belief of many primitive peoples that a child is born because it wants to be. They view a difficult labor as a sign that the child is obstinate and will therefore try to coax it from the mother's body with offers of food or with threats. The unfortunate mother may even be starved to make the child more willing to leave the womb. The fetus's actual role in labor is

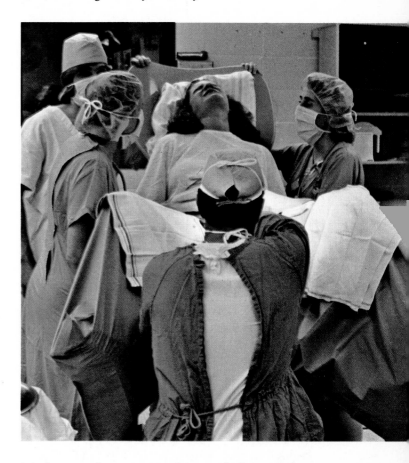

involuntary, but a mature fetus and placenta may start the process by releasing chemical signals. In fetal sheep, labor can be indefinitely postponed when the hypothalamus, the pituitary or both adrenal glands are destroyed. Similarly, delayed labor has been noted in humans when the fetus's pituitary gland is poorly developed.

A woman's body readies itself for labor in a variety of ways. In early pregnancy, the upper portion of the uterus grows heavier and thicker as its cells enlarge. When about 100 times bigger than normal, usually by the fourth month of pregnancy, their growth ceases. The uterine wall is then roughly one centimeter thick — about the width of a paper clip. From then on, the uterus enlarges with the growth of the fetus. Its walls stretch until, shortly before birth, they are only about half that thick. As labor nears, the entrance to the uterus, the cervix, softens. Prelabor contractions gradually cause it to open slightly.

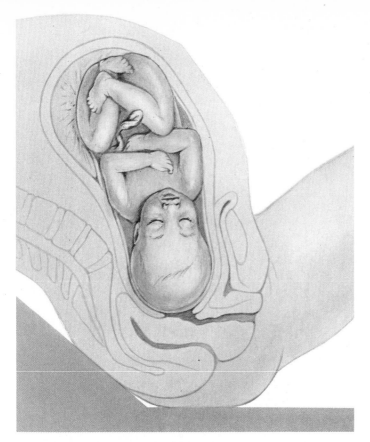
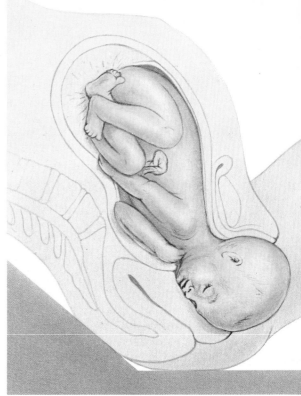

The body sends out signals indicating labor will soon begin. In first pregnancies, the fetus's head will settle into the upper part of the pelvis about two to three weeks before labor. The lower portion of the uterus then expands to accommodate the fetus and the cervix begins to efface, meaning that it is pulled up toward the body of the uterus and dilates. In women who have previously given birth, these events occur much closer to labor or during its early stages.

During pregnancy, a mucous plug forms in the cervix to keep the fetus free from germs. As the cervix grows wider just before labor, the plug usually slips out, tinged with blood. This occurs a few days or sometimes only several hours before labor. With the discharge of the mucous plug, the membranes that surround the fetus and contain the amniotic fluid fill the cervical opening. These two membranes, the amnion and chorion, may rupture before labor begins, releasing the colorless fluid. If so, labor usually follows within twenty-four hours. In most cases, however, the membranes do not rupture until labor has begun.

Labor is a three-stage process. The first comes to an end with the full dilation of the cervix. The delivery of the baby separates the second and third stages, and labor ceases with the expulsion of the afterbirth. The first stage of labor is the longest and the most difficult, taking an average of fourteen hours for women giving birth for the first time and eight hours for women who have had other children. The whole process eases with every birth. A woman who has already had three or four children may be in labor for only an hour. Variations are normal and common, however.

The surest sign of true labor is the arrival of persistent, regular contractions. Contractions are the means by which the uterus opens the cervix and pushes the baby out. Muscle cells of the uterus shorten to create each contraction. When they relax, they do not return to their original size, but remain slightly short of it. Gradually, the cells grow shorter and broader, thickening the uterine wall and reducing its capacity. As uterine capacity falls, the fetus, membranes and fluids are pushed down, forcing the cervix open. The uterus also dilates the cervix by pulling up the cervical walls as it shortens.

The timing and duration of contractions vary from woman to woman. Usually they arrive in twenty-minute intervals and last thirty seconds or so. As labor progresses, the intervals shorten and the contractions last longer. A woman is usually instructed to notify her obstetrician when

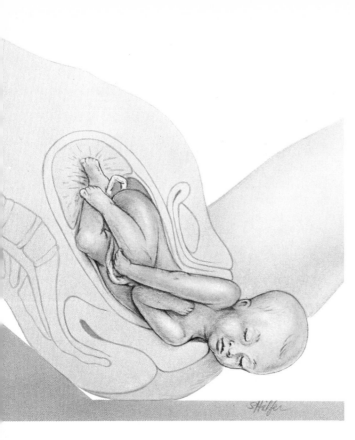

Birth, life's most important journey, is but inches long. The baby must gently twist through the narrow tunnel of his mother's pelvis before making his entrance into the world. Held aloft, the newborn's only remaining physical tie to the womb is the umbilical cord, spiralling down into his mother's body. It continues to send him blood and oxygen in the first moments after birth. Most infants begin the task of breathing on their own in a minute or two.

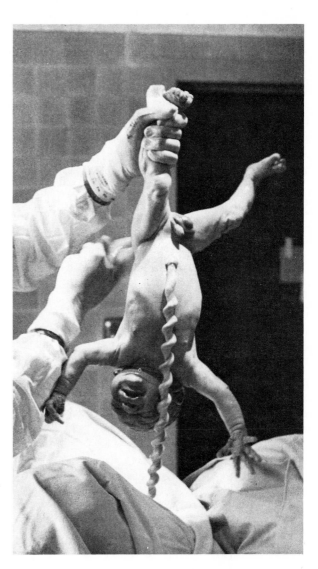

the contractions are eight minutes apart. Eight hours after contractions begin — less in subsequent births — their pace increases to one every five minutes; the cervix is then dilated about three centimeters. While it opens an additional five centimeters, the contractions arrive every two to four minutes, but only last one. As the cervix reaches full dilation — just before an infant is born — contractions are severe, occurring every minute or two and lasting almost as long.

When the cervix fully dilates, about ten centimeters, the second stage of labor begins. This stage can take from two hours to just minutes depending on the number of previous births. As the baby starts moving down the birth canal, the contractions slow down somewhat and the woman can begin to "work" with them. By bearing down her abdominal muscles she can double the force of contraction, exerting sixty pounds of pressure. If the membranes have not ruptured, they soon will. The doctor may also break them to speed labor. When birth takes place in a hospital, the mother is moved into the delivery room shortly before the baby's head is visible.

As the infant's head is about to emerge, the skin of the mother's pelvic floor, the area surrounding the vagina, begins to bulge outward.

Most children are born head first but there are always a few hearty individualists to challenge doctors, as this page from an eighteenth-century encyclopedia shows. These positions increase risk to the baby.

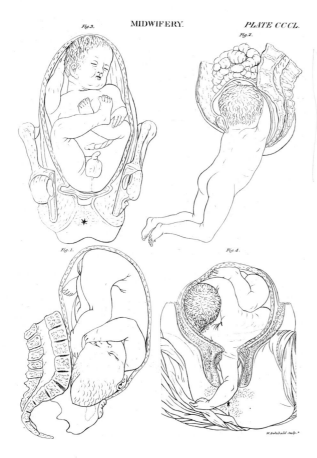

MIDWIFERY. PLATE CCCL.

The mother is asked to cease pushing at this point, for rapid delivery could injure the baby. With each contraction, the head pushes farther and the mother's skin stretches wider. The doctor may perform an episiotomy, a small cut at the base of the vaginal opening, to ease delivery and prevent the mother's skin from tearing.

Because the baby passes through a relatively tight space at birth, its body rotates. The head turns over the shoulder in passage through the pelvis and usually emerges face down but quickly returns to its natural position. If the umbilical cord is wrapped around the baby's neck, which happens in about 25 percent of births, the doctor eases it over the baby's head to prevent strangulation. Like the head, the baby's shoulders must rotate to pass through the mother's pelvis. The doctor will move the baby's head downward slightly to bring one shoulder forward. Then he lifts the head to ease the other shoulder from the

mother's body. Once the head and shoulders have emerged the rest of the birth proceeds rapidly. The baby's body is finally free of its nine-month-long home. The pearly blue umbilical cord still links child to womb, sending him blood from the placenta. The doctor will wait until the cord has stopped pulsating before clamping it above the baby's abdomen and severing it. This does not cause pain to mother or infant because the cord has no nerves.

The uterus continues to contract after the birth of the baby until the placenta is expelled. As the baby is born, the uterus begins to shrink. The placenta will partially or totally separate, usually in the late stages of birth or with the first few contractions after birth. Continued contractions and some bearing-down assistance from the mother force the placenta from the womb. The doctor sometimes assists by pressing her abdomen. A small gush of blood accompanies delivery of the placenta. Uterine arteries open into cavities in the mucous lining beneath the placenta. As the placenta peels away, its interior pockets release blood, which drains away. The uterus protects against excessive bleeding with firm contractions that compress the open blood vessels, allowing clots to form. After the placenta is delivered, the doctor will examine it to make sure it is intact. It is then discarded or sold to companies for use in research or beauty products.

In other cultures, disposal of the placenta is surrounded in ritual. According to Vietnamese custom, it is buried immediately after birth. The spot is carefully selected, for the people believe a variety of ills might befall a child, all of which can be read from the condition of the placenta. In northern Vietnam, they often place a clay pot containing the placenta on the roof of the house to protect the child from supernatural enemies. Filipinos, too, see a sympathetic relationship between baby and placenta. The Caticugans of the Philippines say that when a father buries the placenta, the bond with his child is strengthened. He buries it deeply lest a dog or pig unearth it, which would make the child a wanderer when he grows up. In America, ritual tends to accompany home births; families often bury the placenta, feeling it too significant to be thrown away.

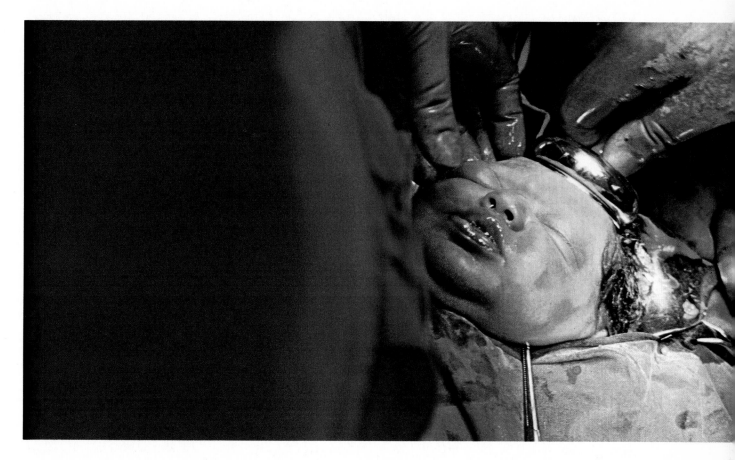

The biology of childbirth has rituals of its own and it also has exceptions. Ninety-five percent of all infants are born head first in a vertex presentation. The head is called the presenting part, meaning simply that it emerges first. In a breech delivery, a little more than 3 percent of all births, the baby's position in the womb is reversed, with buttocks or legs presenting. In a full breech, the baby is in a squatting position in the womb, knees drawn up to its chest. In a frank breech, the most common breech, the baby's body flexes at the hips rather than the knees, as though it has been folded in half. In an incomplete breech, one or both feet or one or both knees are presenting.

A Surgical Alternative

The fetal mortality from breech births is three times higher than in vertex deliveries. Injuries are more frequent because of the necessary added manipulation. A procedure known as version can be employed to change a fetus's position in the womb, but its uses are limited. The doctor can manipulate the fetus externally, but never when the patient is in labor. Internal version is used only in the second stage of labor to move the baby from a vertex or shoulder presentation so that he can be extracted by the feet. This is generally done only to deliver a second twin or to remove a dead fetus. Vaginal deliveries are possible in many breech presentations, but doctors tend to opt for delivery by caesarean section, which they feel is safer for the infant.

Caesarean section is the delivery of the fetus through an incision in the mother's abdomen and uterus. Only in relatively recent times has it become a safe, widespread procedure. According to legend, Julius Caesar was cut from his mother's womb. Both his name and the operation may derive from the same Latin root — the verb *caedere,* meaning "to cut." In all likelihood, however, the

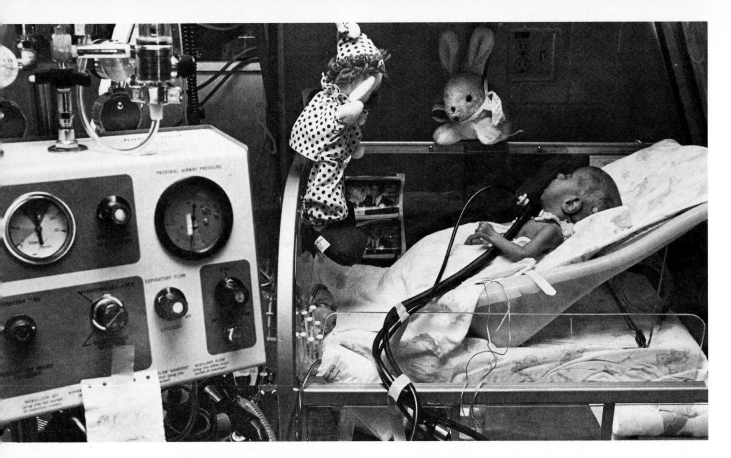

Roman emperor was probably not delivered by caesarean for there is evidence that his mother lived well after his birth, a virtual impossibility given the procedure of the times.

According to a law initiated in eighth-century Rome and carried through the Middle Ages, a woman who died in childbirth could not be buried unless the child was taken from her body and baptized. A few accounts of caesareans performed on living women began to appear during the Renaissance. The operations were performed without anesthesia but the author of the first guide to caesarean surgery, which was published in Paris in 1581, reasoned that the pain of the operation would be less than the pain of futile labor. As was later discovered, the author, surgeon François Rousset, had never performed a caesarean and might never have witnessed one. Perhaps well-intentioned, the work could only have added to mortality figures. But tales of remarkably early successes also exist. In 1500, a Swiss butcher, unable to stand the agony of his wife's prolonged labor, cut the child from her womb and saved both lives. The child thrived, according to the storyteller, living to be seventy-seven years old. And the mother, having miraculously survived the operation, went on to give

birth normally to five more children. A more realistic account describes a caesarean performed by a German surgeon who delivered a live infant in 1610. The mother, however, did not survive.

Today, caesarean delivery has become so safe that its practice has increased dramatically. Aside from the majority of breech births, the procedure is used as an alternative to prolonged, difficult labor. Caesareans are performed when the baby's head is too large to pass through its mother's pelvis, if the baby's oxygen supply might drop or if normal delivery would threaten the life of the baby or mother in any way. Fifteen to 20 percent of deliveries are caesarean, a figure three times higher than in the 1960s.

The greatest single factor contributing to the high incidence of caesareans is the long-accepted dictum "once a caesarean, always a caesarean." Doctors used to fear that vaginal deliveries would rupture the caesarean scar. A recent review of studies of more than 28,000 vaginal deliveries following caesareans indicates that this is not necessarily true. In early 1982, the American College of Obstetricians and Gynecologists concluded that many women who have had caesareans can safely undergo subsequent vaginal deliveries. However safe caesareans have be-

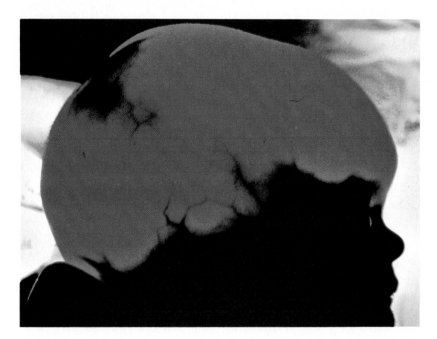

come, they remain major surgery and should be avoided if unnecessary. Nature's way of birth is still the best.

Born Too Soon

Occasionally, Nature needs a little help. The greatest strides in the science of birth have been in the care and treatment of premature babies, those born before the full-term, thirty-seventh week of pregnancy. Today, such infants survive and thrive. Often, a little more than a decade ago, premature babies had a slim chance of doing so.

Many factors seem to contribute to premature labor. Twins and triplets are often born early because the uterus reaches full extension sooner than usual. If the membranes rupture too soon, labor will begin, but it is still uncertain why this happens. The placement and condition of the placenta also appear to affect premature labor. If the placenta attaches to the uterus at the point of dilation — above the cervix — or when it separates early, labor usually begins. If the placenta begins to separate and labor does not proceed, the doctor will induce contractions to save the baby. Premature labor may also result from an abnormal uterus. High blood pressure, sometimes occurring in late pregnancy, and diabetes are also thought to be factors. Cigarette smoking has been linked to premature labor and undersized infants. For most premature births, however, doctors are unable to find an explanation.

Prematurity is the leading cause of baby deaths in the United States. As one doctor succinctly put it, premature birth is as much a surprise for the baby as it is for the mother. It may be outside the womb, but a very early "preemie" is really still a fetus. Its skin is fragile and wrinkled because it lacks the underlying layer of fat that later develops and it is covered with the downy hair that normally disappears during the last few weeks of the fetus's development.

The greatest challenge in treating premature infants lies in balancing their support systems. Doctors must struggle to keep a preemie's artificial maintenance systems from adversely affecting its underdeveloped body. Intensive care units for newborns are a touching blend of the technological world of the scientist and the poignant, innocent world of the child. Taped inside their Isolettes, the artificial "wombs" that keep newborns in a regulated environment, are pictures of the parents. Floppy stuffed animals lying next to the babies are a sharp contrast to the lights, tubes and wires of life-sustaining, intensive care.

The world is a hazardous place for these infants. Their lungs, the last organs to develop before a baby is born, are immature. Doctors now have a variety of methods to sustain a preemie's breathing. The lungs' degree of maturity in the womb can be tested to determine how well they will be able to stand up to the rigors of birth. If the results are discouraging, doctors can administer hormones to a woman in premature labor to stimulate development of the fetus's lungs. Once the baby is born, ventilating machines deliver air to the tiny, fragile lungs.

But these babies also face a host of problems that do not have ready solutions. Their hearts usually function inefficiently, tending to bypass the lungs — normal procedure when the child is still in the womb. Half of the premature infants weighing under 3.3 pounds suffer from brain hemorrhaging, bleeding under the skull, which claims many lives. Such hemorrhaging may have a lingering effect on infants who survive severe bleeding episodes, leaving them with neurological disorders. A premature baby's eyes are also in great danger; their fragile blood vessels are highly susceptible to increases in the oxygen level of the baby's blood. When treating premature infants, doctors must consider oxygen a drug to be used sparingly and monitored carefully. Both doctors and parents may still be faced with the decision of sacrificing an infant's sight to save his life if his need for oxygen exceeds the level that is safe for his eyes.

Researchers are also investigating the possible psychological damage that premature babies may suffer from spending their first weeks in intensive care. Premature birth certainly affects the mother. Such mothers often say they have feelings of unreality after giving birth sooner than expected. Even though they have gone through months of pregnancy and have experienced labor, they still do not feel like mothers. They find themselves worrying incessantly over an alarmingly tiny and quiet baby who needs constant attention and assistance merely to survive. A sense of guilt is common; many preemie mothers think they have failed their babies in some way.

Because premature deliveries are so traumatic, doctors delay labor when possible. Simple bed rest, an old-fashioned treatment, tends to delay labor, especially in multiple pregnancies. A more modern treatment shows great promise. In mid-1980, the U. S. Food and Drug Administration approved ritodrine hydrochloride, a drug that relaxes the uterus and thus prevents contractions. Doctors recommend its use during labor when prematurity seems to be the only complication. The drug also proved successful in prolonging one multiple pregnancy. In mid-1981, a woman carrying triplets went into labor in her twenty-seventh week of pregnancy — more than two months early. Doctors, knowing the chances of her babies' survival were slim if labor continued, used ritodrine to halt contractions. On two later occasions, they again administered the drug when contractions began. Five weeks after her first contractions had started, three healthy boys were born. The mother then faced the comparatively pleasant problem of how she would tell her babies apart.

Extra Heartbeats

One of the greatest surprises to greet an expectant mother is the news that she is carrying more than one baby. A doctor should be able to detect multiple fetuses within the first three months of pregnancy through ultrasound, a technological procedure using sound waves to create images of the uterus's contents. X-ray diagnosis of multiple pregnancy is possible by the sixth month. A doctor may also be able to tell by probing the surface of the mother's abdomen with his fingers or listening for extra heartbeats, but these methods are not as accurate.

When a multiple pregnancy has been determined, the mother requires special attention. Carrying more than one baby puts a measurable strain on her body. The usual aches and pains of pregnancy are greater. Morning sickness will be more severe and will last longer. The added weight contributes to more varicose veins and hemorrhoids and to more severe backaches and pelvic pressure. A multiple pregnancy also causes the cervix to dilate sooner. Indeed, premature labor poses the biggest hazard. A physician usually counsels the mother not to travel in the last few months and may suggest bed rest.

By the time the mother goes into labor, the doctor should have an accurate idea of the babies' positions. Delivery of the second baby is usually more complicated than the first. When the first is delivered, the doctor will immediately try to determine the position of the second baby because it may have shifted while its sibling was being born. If the second baby is lying sideways in the womb, the doctor will try to rotate it for delivery, head or buttocks first. Speed is necessary. The placenta may well separate from the uterus after the first birth, endangering the second baby. In multiple births, babies are often smaller than those of single pregnancies, but they catch up quickly.

For all its joy, childbirth has a long association with pain, a complex sensation that scientists do not fully understand. Childbirth is even more perplexing because it is a rare instance of pain accompanying a normal function. The word *pain* has its origins in the Greek and Latin words meaning "penalty," a connotation elaborated on in the Bible. For having tasted the forbidden apple, Eve was to suffer punishments, among them one that countless generations of women would inherit: "... in sorrow thou shalt bring forth children ." In Europe, common belief held that pain accompanied childbirth because God had ruled it so. Little was done, therefore, to relieve it. In sixteenth-century Scotland, an Edinburgh midwife was burned at the stake after giving painkilling medicine to a woman in labor. Some two centuries later, the same Scottish city was the scene of another event that would change the conventional wisdom.

A Curse Conquered

Scottish obstetrician James Simpson regularly experimented with painkilling drugs which he hoped to use in his work. He had already worked with ether but hoped to find a more satisfactory drug. In 1847, Simpson met with two colleagues to test chloroform, a drug that had recently come to their attention. One of the first people to hear of the experiment was James Miller, a surgeon, friend and neighbor of Simpson's. As Miller later recorded the evening's happenings, the three doctors "sat down to their somewhat hazardous

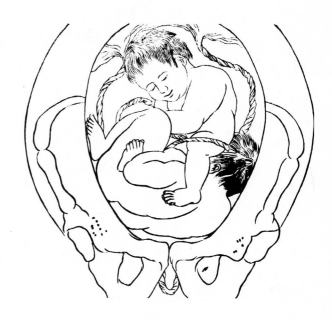

Japanese twins frolic in the womb in this print from a nineteenth-century midwifery manual. Twins occur about once in every ninety pregnancies in the United States, but among orientals they are much more rare.

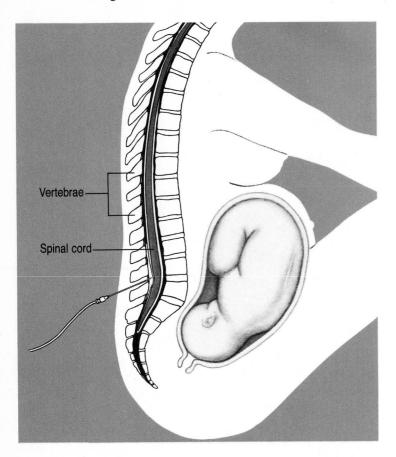

Vertebrae

Spinal cord

work in Dr. Simpson's dining room." With their first inhalation, "an unwonted hilarity seized the party; they became bright-eyed, very happy, and very loquacious, expatiating on the delicious aroma of the new fluid. The conversation was of unusual intelligence, and quite charmed the listeners." The experiment climaxed in noisy confusion before all succumbed to the fumes. "On awakening, Dr. Simpson's first perception was mental: 'this is far stronger and better than ether,' he said to himself. His second was to note that he was prostrate to the floor." So were his assistants. Gradually, the doctors returned to their seats at the table. "Each expressed himself delighted with this new agent, and its inhalation was repeated many times that night . . . until the supply of chloroform was fairly exhausted."

Soon thereafter, Simpson used chloroform on a patient. The woman, Jane Carstairs, had dreaded this birth. Her previous pregnancy ended in three days of agonizing labor, leaving her with a stillborn child. Simpson moistened a handkerchief with chloroform and held it over his patient's nose. About twenty-five minutes later, a daughter was born. The birth had proceeded so effortlessly that the doctor had trouble convincing Mrs. Carstairs that it was over and that the healthy, cleaned and wrapped child was her own.

Within days, Simpson had used chloroform in about fifty cases and was convinced that it was an ideal anesthetic. In promoting its benefits, Simpson met immediate opposition. A leading Irish obstetrician disapproved of anesthesia "merely to avert the ordinary amount of pain, which the Almighty had seen fit — and most wisely, no doubt — to allot to natural labour." Simpson responded in parody: "I do not believe that anyone in Dublin has yet used a carriage in locomotion; the feeling is very strong against its use in ordinary progression, merely to avert the ordinary amount of fatigue which the Almighty has seen fit — and most wisely no doubt — to [allot to] natural walking." For doctors who questioned the safety of anesthesia, he produced figures showing a higher survival rate for patients given painkillers. And for those doctors who turned to the biblical account of Eve's punishment in arguing against the use of anesthetics, Simpson had ready another quotation from the Book of Genesis in which God, before removing one of Adam's ribs to create Eve, "caused a deep sleep to fall upon Adam."

The idea of relieving pain in childbirth was introduced in the United States one year after Simpson's experiment with chloroform. In 1848, Boston obstetrician Walter Channing published *A Treatise on Etherization in Childbirth,* in which he systematically outlined arguments in favor of painkillers, tackling the same issues Simpson had. Channing wrote of one patient who "with an expression of bodily agony and mental terror, exclaimed, 'I am scared!' and became at once still as if death had taken place." He had "never witnessed such suffering, nor have I ever witnessed such an expression of it."

The most convincing argument championing anesthesia did not come from either Simpson or Channing, but from Queen Victoria. In 1853, the queen chose to receive chloroform when she gave birth to her eighth child, Leopold. Although critics continued to denounce the practice, its popularity quickly grew.

In 1907, a German doctor transformed the use of painkillers in childbirth into a procedure given the soothing name "twilight sleep." When labor began, a woman was first given morphine, a thought- and sensation-numbing drug extracted from poppies, and scopolamine, a drug that induced temporary amnesia. Just before delivery, ether or chloroform tackled the remaining pain. Painless childbirth had an obvious appeal. The technique, arising with the feminist movement, quickly caught on in America. In her 1927 novel, *Twilight Sleep,* Edith Wharton created a character, Lita, who gives birth with painkillers: "All she asked was that nothing should 'hurt' her: she had the blind dread of physical pain common also to most of the young women of her set. But all that was so easily managed nowadays ... and Lita drifted into motherhood as lightly and unperceivingly as if the wax doll which suddenly appeared in the cradle at her bedside had been brought there in one of the big bunches of hothouse roses that she found every morning on her pillow." By the 1930s, the procedure became a firmly established hospital routine and helped to make hospitals a safe place for all births.

Today, there are a variety of techniques available to relieve the pain of labor. But none is ideal. Any painkiller in the mother's blood stream will eventually reach the fetus, possibly endangering its immature nervous system. Doctors try to reach the delicate balance between maximum relief for the mother and minimal danger to the fetus. There is also danger in the drug's interfering with the expulsive efforts of the uterus. For this reason, painkillers are usually not administered until labor is well established.

Two major classes of pain relievers, analgesics and anesthetics, are used in childbirth to inhibit the sensation of pain. The most commonly administered analgesic for labor pain in the United States is meperidine hydrochloride, better known as Demerol. General anesthesia, which renders a patient unconscious, is usually administered only during complicated labor or at delivery.

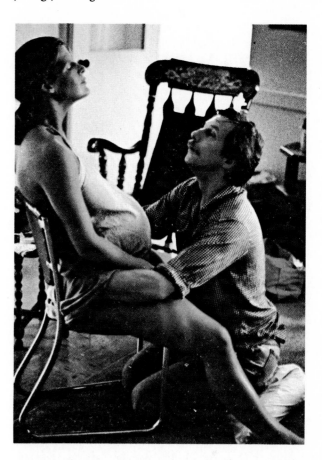

Regional anesthesia has recently gained popularity because it allows the mother to remain conscious during the birth. The most popular and the most widely favored by doctors is the continuous lumbar epidural block. To administer an epidural, an anesthesiologist inserts a needle between two of the patient's lumbar vertebrae in the lower back. The needle opens near the spinal cord. A thin plastic tube, threaded through the needle, carries a constant, measured supply of anesthesia. The epidural is continuously administered, usually midway through labor to the repair of lacerations immediately after birth.

Nature Reevaluated

Just as twilight sleep was gaining acceptance, work was already under way which would move childbirth away from a reliance on painkillers. In the 1920s, British obstetrician Grantly Dick-Read assisted a woman giving birth in Whitechapel, a

105

poor, working-class area of London. The dark, run-down room admitted the pouring rain from outside, but the patient seemed comfortable and the labor progressed smoothly. He offered her chloroform but, to his surprise, she refused it. When the child was born, the woman looked shyly at the doctor and said, "It didn't hurt. It wasn't meant to, was it, doctor?"

For months, Dick-Read found himself thinking about the woman's words. He came "to realize there was no law in nature and no design that could justify the pain of childbirth." Most childbirth pain must be culturally learned, he reasoned, and could be alleviated if women better understood the birth process and learned methods of relaxation. With the publication of *Natural Childbirth* in England in 1933, and in America in 1944 as *Childbirth Without Fear*, Dick-Read offered women an alternative and began what is now called the natural childbirth movement.

The movement gained momentum through the work of a French obstetrician, Fernand Lamaze. In 1951, Lamaze, who described himself as an "elderly schoolboy of sixty," visited the Soviet Union to study a newly developed and nationally instituted technique of childbirth. The method, given the burdensome name psychoprophylaxis, utilizes the simple will power of a woman to psychologically master pain. Women learn to respond to contractions with measured, rhythmic breathing that provides a focus for concentration and supplements the body's increased oxygen demand during the strenuous process of labor.

When Lamaze watched a Russian woman who had been trained in the psychoprophylactic method give birth with no evidence of pain, he found the spectacle so inspiring that he instituted the practice, with a few minor changes, in his maternity clinic in Paris. About eight years later, in 1959, the method spread to the United States with the publication of *Thank You, Dr. Lamaze,* an American woman's enthusiastic endorsement of his work. Lamaze claimed that his method could eliminate pain completely without the use of any drugs. He died in 1957 just as his ideas were gaining wide acceptance in childbirth.

Preparation for the Lamaze method of birth usually begins in the woman's seventh month of pregnancy. Taught the basic physiology and biology of pregnancy and birth, she rehearses breathing patterns and exercises to condition her body for labor. Soon, the regulated breathing becomes second nature. The mother is also taught *effleurage,* the gentle fingertip massage of her abdomen, to relax the muscles of the abdominal wall and provide her with another point of mental concentration. Assistants are instructed to maintain a calm, supportive atmosphere during labor and delivery.

Recent studies evaluating the success rate of prepared childbirth training have demonstrated that women who participate in childbirth training experience significantly lower levels of pain than women who have no training. But the reduction of pain is not as dramatic as the title of Lamaze's book, *Painless Childbirth,* suggests. One Canadian study, conducted at McGill University, revealed that 81 percent of women who had had prepared childbirth training requested epidural anesthesia when giving birth. Many of these women felt that by requesting a painkiller, they had failed themselves. The researchers concluded that while the benefits of prepared childbirth training are incontestable, the classes should also train expectant mothers in anesthetic procedures they might elect during labor.

Sometimes, the mother is not the only member of the family who feels the pains of childbirth. In certain primitive cultures, when the mother is in labor, the father takes to bed. Shortly after birth, she will resume work but he will remain in bed with the child. Anthropologists, fascinated by couvade, as this ritual is called, offer a variety of hypotheses for its existence. Predominantly, they believe the father's false labor is thought to lure bad spirits away from the mother as she gives birth. Some anthropologists suggest that couvade is not conscious play-acting but is an expression of the father's actual feeling of pain.

Couvade is a widespread phenomenon. In modern America, fathers-to-be routinely fall victim to low back pain, cramps and morning sickness when their wives are pregnant. These aches and pains appear to follow a pattern, generally arriving in the wife's third month of pregnancy. They subside and then flare up again in her ninth month or at the time of labor. The most frequent symptoms of this syndrome are loss of appetite, toothaches, nausea or vomiting and abdominal colic. One researcher estimated about one in nine men suffers from some sort of empathetic pain.

Such empathy for a woman's experience is, on occasion, the subject of jokes just as the mother's pains are matter for legend. But what about the baby? French obstetrician Frederick Leboyer believes the baby's introduction to the world is one of trauma. The idea of birth trauma is not new. Otto Rank, a disciple of Sigmund Freud, believed that all anxiety and neuroses could be traced to birth. *The Trauma of Birth,* which he published in 1923, forms the basic principles that underlie several modern psychotherapies, such as rebirthing, in which the subject reenacts birth and thereby presumably erases its anxieties. Leboyer was first to propose that steps could be taken to spare the infant this initial trauma.

Leboyer's ideas were presented in *Birth Without Violence,* an emotional book published in 1974. "Poor little creature!" he wrote. "What a fate, to be born and to fall into our hands, victim of our ignorance and cruelty!" His suggestions, rather simple, were quickly adopted. To shield a baby's unaccustomed eyes, the intense lighting of the delivery room should be dimmed. Similarly, voices should be hushed. When a baby is born, Leboyer favors placing it immediately on the mother's stomach so that she can help keep it warm and comforted. The umbilical cord is not immediately severed. Nor is the infant immediately weighed or bundled up; it is given time to adjust to its new environment. To help it do so, the baby is immersed in a tub of water warmed to body temperature until it seems relaxed and happy. Then the baby is wrapped in soft fabric and again given to its mother, placed on its side rather than its back so that the spine which has been curved for so many months in the womb is not suddenly straightened.

A Measure of Health

Each newborn undergoes standard tests after birth to make sure it is healthy. The first series of tests is carried out immediately in the delivery room, where the nurse quickly assesses the

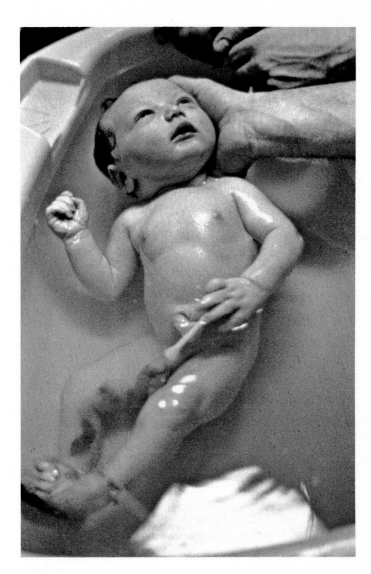

Weightless in warm water, a baby relaxes only minutes after birth. French obstetrician Frederick Leboyer believes a bath simulates the womb and helps the baby adjust in his strange, new world.

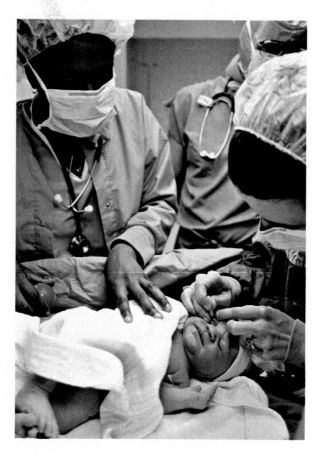

A delivery-room nurse places silver nitrate drops in a newborn's eyes. Required by law in most states, the treatment protects the eyes from a gonorrheal infection. The drops may cause a temporary irritation.

baby's physical condition, using the Apgar scoring system. To ensure accuracy, the Apgar evaluations are made twice, one minute and five minutes after birth. The nurse checks five categories and assigns a score ranging from zero to two for each test. A perfect Apgar score is ten, which is unusual. Infants with scores below six will require some sort of resuscitation. Heartbeat is normally 120 to 150 beats per minute, although it may rise as high as 200 if the baby is crying. If the rate is less than 100 beats per minute, the baby needs immediate resuscitation. Next, the baby's breathing, muscle tone and reflex irritability (determined by poking the soles of its feet) are checked. Finally, the color of the infant's skin is inspected to make sure that the baby is getting enough oxygen. Most babies have a blue tinge in their limbs, a normal coloration that disappears in a few minutes.

The nurse may next administer one or two drops of silver nitrate solution to the infant's eyes. This treatment is required by law in most states to protect against a gonorrheal infection of the eyes that can be picked up in the birth canal and lead to blindness. Because the treatment may cause a slight irritation, some obstetricians recommend that it be postponed until the baby has had a chance to adjust to his new environment. Before sending the baby to the nursery, the nurse makes sure there are no physical deformities that need immediate attention.

A more detailed physical that follows is carried out in the nursery. The nurse weighs the baby and takes a variety of measurements, such as the size of the fontanelles, the places in its skull not yet filled in by hard bone. Likewise, physical symmetry of face and limbs are noted. Lastly, the baby's nervous system is evaluated by reviewing certain reflexes common to the newborn. The rooting reflex ensures that the baby will be able to search out its mother's nipple to nurse. To test this reflex, the nurse puts a finger at the side of the baby's mouth or near its cheek. The baby should turn its head and open its mouth, trying to suck the finger. Touching the baby's palm with a finger should elicit the grasp reflex, a firm grip by the tiny hand. With the stepping reflex, an infant held upright with one foot touching the table should be able to lift and place its feet as if trying to walk. This reflex is pronounced at birth but disappears after the baby is two months old.

An infant unhappy with these strange proceedings will probably respond by crying and this, too, the nurse assesses. A strong, lusty cry is a sign of a healthy baby. Abnormalities in the cry may indicate neurological disorders. Crying is the baby's only tool of communication. Infants as young as eight weeks old are capable of recognizing that they can get what they want by crying. Ann M. Frodi, a researcher at the University of Rochester in New York, thinks that Nature intended a baby's cry to be irritating. She measured the physiological responses of children and adults to the sound of an infant's cry and found them to be nearly identical. Frodi thinks crying is a survival mechanism, meant to motivate comforting the infant and providing it with what it needs. She also noted that premature and malnourished babies cry an octave higher than fullterm babies and that the cries have a different rhythm and pattern, increasing the irritant effect.

The baby also shapes his world by crying and draws conclusions about that world based on how parents respond to the cries. If comforted, the baby will feel secure. But if the cries go unanswered, the baby may give up hope and withdraw. Some doctors say that a baby may need to cry, perhaps fifteen minutes every day, just for crying's sake, to help relieve sensory "overload." To those who can read it, an infant's cry is an expressive language all its own.

Baby Blues

Like the newborn, the new mother's first days and weeks after birth are likely to be confusing. She may feel moody, easily upset and irritable. These "baby blues" are called postpartum depression. The blues usually strike about three days after delivery, when the mother starts giving milk — timing that suggests the depression may have hormonal roots. But its other causes are more obvious and probably more important. Her life has changed, and she faces new responsibilities. She and her body have been through a great deal of stress and both are still suffering from it. Some depression is normal.

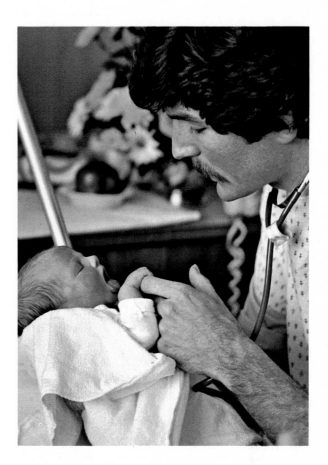

With a blasé air, a premature baby demonstrates a basic reflex in grasping his doctor's finger. Infants are born with a variety of reflexes linked to their instinct for survival, all indicating neurological health.

109

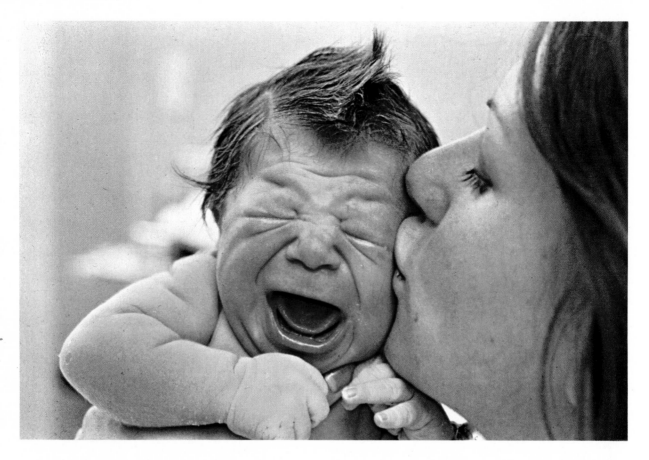

Her body will continue to change after birth. Following delivery of the baby and placenta, the mother's uterus rapidly shrinks. The reduction continues during the next few weeks, primarily caused by the shrinking of the uterine muscle cells. Six weeks after birth, the uterus will have returned to its prepregnancy size. The cervix, too, starts firming and constricting. One week after it admitted a baby into the world, its opening is only one or two centimeters wide. The vagina, too, shrinks rapidly, but neither it nor the cervix will ever return to their original size. The mother's abdominal wall remains flabby until the muscles regain their tone. Exercises, like leg lifts and sit-ups, help firm up muscle long stretched.

The mother's breasts, which expanded during pregnancy, will feel large, heavy and tender as they ready for feeding her baby. Female hormones promote breast growth during pregnancy but inhibit the production of milk. Once the baby is born, the hormonal barrier breaks down, probably facilitated by the expulsion of the placenta. The pituitary increases its secretion of the hormone prolactin, which stimulates milk production. Oxytocin, the hormone that also acts as a uterine stimulant, contributes to milk production by permitting the movement of milk into pockets in the breast where it is stored.

The mother's milk flow usually begins a few days after birth, although she will secrete a substance called colostrum for the first few days. This works out fine for the infant, who tends to fast, or nearly so, the first day after birth. Healthy babies normally lose about one-tenth of their birth weight in this period. In the meantime, the colostrum, a yellowish liquid, provides the baby with protein and antibodies and acts as a laxative. Once milk begins to flow, the baby's suckling increases the production and flow by stimulating the release of prolactin and oxytocin.

The closer scientists examine human milk, the more remarkable a substance it appears to be. Its role is much more complex than nourishment, although in that, too, it excels. A mother's milk is rich in macrophages, fierce defenders against infection. A breast-fed baby also receives antibodies to help its developing immune system fight infection. The baby already has some antibodies from its mother, which it retains for several months to a year after birth. Antibodies present in the milk protect the baby from intestinal infection, a common affliction of newborns. The milk also speeds the maturation of the infant's immune system. Breast-fed babies are known to be more resistant to general infection and allergies than bottle-fed babies.

A Lasting Bond

Breast-feeding has psychological as well as physical benefits. Newborns need to continue close contact with their mothers. History records that Frederick II, Holy Roman Emperor and king of Germany and Sicily in the thirteenth century, conducted an experiment to determine which language was innate to man. He ordered mothers and nurses not to talk to or play with their infants so that the babies would be free of outside influence. But the experiment was never completed — all the children died.

Human infants crave love almost as much as they crave warmth, comfort and food. And it is just as important for their development. What sensitive mothers have known for ages has recently been investigated by science. In the early 1970s, pediatricians John Kennell and Marshall Klaus of the Case Western Reserve School of Medicine in Cleveland reported their observations of a process they called "bonding." The researchers concluded that "there is a sensitive period in the first minutes and hours after the infant's birth which is optimal for infant-parent attachment." Babies spend about the first forty minutes of life in a state of watchful awareness, a state the pediatricians believe may facilitate bonding between child and parents. Kennell and Klaus noticed that mothers allowed to spend this time with their infants as well as about five hours over each of the next few days, behaved

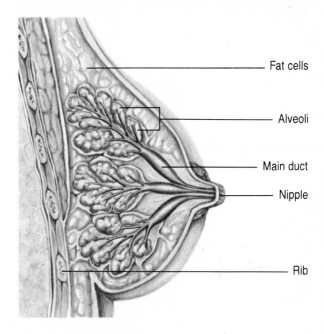

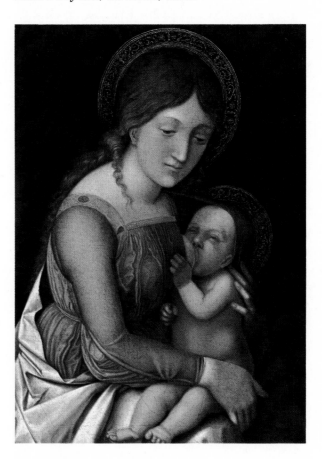

Fat cells

Alveoli

Main duct

Nipple

Rib

*"Love comes in at the eye," penned
William Butler Yeats. This infant's
gaze seems determined to capture it.
From their first hour, babies prime
their senses in wide-eyed wonder,
alertly surveying the surroundings.*

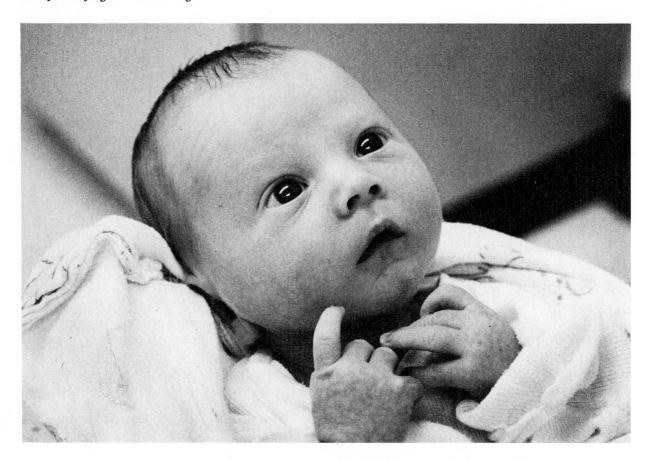

*An infant listens to a recording of
his mother's voice by sucking on a
nipple at a fixed rate. If he alters the
sucking pattern, he hears another
woman's voice, not nearly as soothing as his mother's. Doctors have
found that a baby strives to prevent
the change, maintaining the pattern
for intervals all day.*

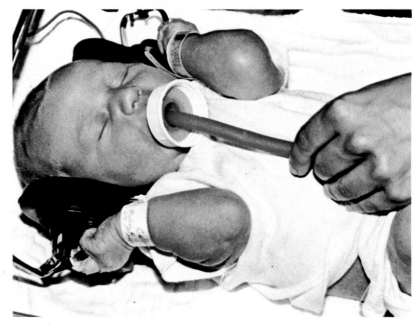

A carefree romp between father and son helps establish a loving bond. More and more, psychologists are discovering that the way to healthy mental development for a baby is — quite literally — child's play.

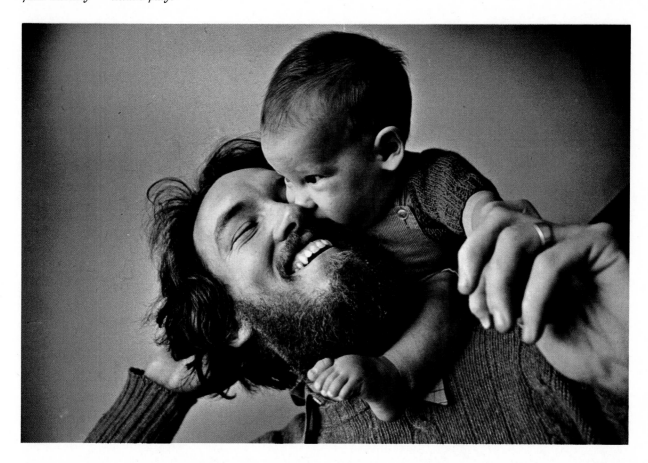

differently toward their children than mothers not permitted to spend time with their babies. Kennell and Klaus suggest that this initial contact influences the behavior of mother and infant for months and years to come. Follow-up studies indicated that babies allowed to stay with mothers after birth were physically healthier and had higher IQs and that the mothers were more affectionate and responsive. Critics, while applauding the doctors' emphasis on physical contact after birth, emphasize that it is not essential to the formation of close and lasting ties.

There is a growing realization that human infants are intelligent, capable of learning and responding in their first hours of life. Less than 100 years ago, J. P. C. Griffith counseled mothers that the newborn baby was "very little more intelligent than a vegetable." Researchers have discovered that quite the opposite is true. Within the first hour after birth, a baby's eyes are wide open

and alert, searching out the sources of sounds. The newborn shows a preference for human voices over other sounds, female voices over male voices and its mother's voice above all others. Babies' sensitivity to human voices was studied on film by two psychiatrists who discovered, by slowing down the film, that infants moved their bodies in synchrony with voices they heard.

Babies also appear to respond to different behavior. A researcher at the Children's Hospital Medical Center in Boston noticed that infants several weeks old are more playful and alert with the more playful of their parents. By shaping responses to the surroundings and tailoring behavior to others, babies begin to master subtleties of human interaction. The birth of a child signals the arrival of more than one new identity in the world. The wife becomes a mother, the husband a father. Together, they forge a new bond, one as timeless but ever-changing as birth itself.

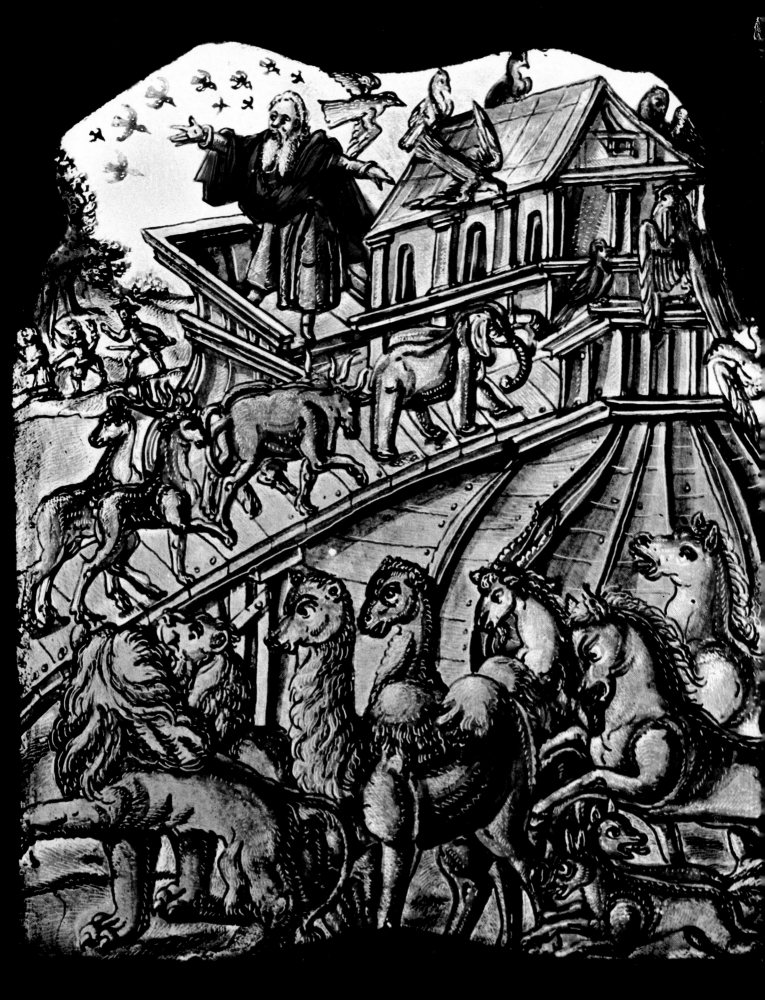

Chapter 5

An Elusive Balance

When American author Moritz Thomsen was stationed with the Peace Corps in Ecuador in the late 1960s, he arrived one morning at a small rural school to keep a rendezvous with some of the local farmers. They were going to clear a garden out of the jungle, a standard project aimed at bringing a few fresh vegetables to the hungry people of a Third World village. Many of the farmers' families came to watch. Among them was a mother holding an infant that was writhing in agony, sputtering and gasping for breath through the foam of advanced pneumonia. All along, there had been a doctor nearby who might have saved the child's life, but the family had waited too long. They gathered round and watched with a detachment that infuriated Thomsen. Only the mother seemed upset by the ordeal. Thomsen knew the philosophy: the child would die, be released from a life of poverty and suffering and fly directly to heaven to become one of God's *angelitos*. It was a blessing to the family. He knew the statistics, too: in the rural areas of Ecuador, three in every five babies died before their third year. "But," as he would recall in *Living Poor*, "knowing all this I still could not accept it; it was just too sinfully irrational." Thomsen spent the next four years trying to help the people of Rio Verde hack through the voracious jungles and their own even more unyielding superstitions. Like three-fourths of the world's population, they were tied to an agricultural way of life, in which, during the best of times, only basic needs are satisfied. Although more than half the infants died before the age of three, the overall population continued to grow at an appalling, unmanageable rate. Thomsen had learned the most tragic lesson the Third World teaches: as human life outgrows its resources, the value and dignity of the individual diminish. In many poor nations, the stork still flies ahead of the plow.

Genesis records that "wickedness" abounded when "men began to multiply on the face of the earth." Locked in timeless procession at the Church of St. Michael and Our Lady in Yorkshire, England, the chosen progenitors of generations to come take shelter aboard Noah's ark. Introduced into favorable climes, human numbers multiply with astonishing profligacy.

More than one "lover of populous pavements" swarms through Walt Whitman's city, Manhattan, to celebrate Earth Week in 1970. Measuring success in numbers, man has become a star overnight.

Unchanged in principle for millennia, ancient farming techniques from a fifteenth-century Italian fresco, right, draw from the earth the bounty that sustains the festival of human life.

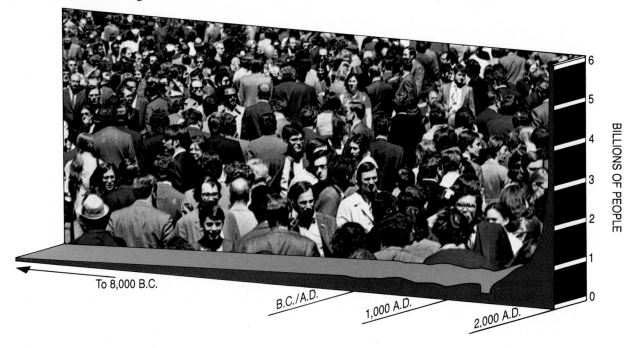

To 8,000 B.C.

B.C./A.D.

1,000 A.D.

2,000 A.D.

BILLIONS OF PEOPLE

6
5
4
3
2
1
0

Many statesmen, economists and social scientists view unabated population growth as the common thread to the world's most urgent problems. Nature imposes limits on all her populations — withholding resources, limiting space, striking through disease and cataclysm with the ferocity of a predator. As a general rule in the animal kingdom, births compensate deaths: they hover on a seesaw, fluctuating but balanced. Through technology and medicine, *Homo sapiens,* man the Wise, seems to have almost broken free of the rule. Plummeting death rates have upset the balance. Today, 115 babies are born every half minute. In the same 30 seconds, there are 45 deaths. One hundred forty people are added to the world's population every minute. In a year's time, the number is approximately equivalent to the total population of Nigeria, the tenth most populous nation in the world. One biologist, looking at a chart of world population growth, was reminded of a graph tracking the advance of a deadly virus in a patient.

Today there is no aspect of population control that escapes controversy. To discuss it is to take aim at the very institutions that have ensured our survival — the family, the bond between mother and child, the instinctual impulse to protect the young and helpless, the sanctity of life. Our reproductive ability is, at best, prolific. At worst, it is dangerously so.

In the story of man, all this has happened overnight. For 99 percent of our existence, for the millions of years before 8000 B.C., man lived a brief, arduous life. Roaming a violent landscape in small and scattered clans, he hunted what game he could, scavenging from the kills of more adept predators, and gathered herbs, berries, roots, wild honey and nuts. There was no crowding. Anthropologists estimate that the population density was low: about one person per ten square kilometers. Few people lived past their fourth decade. With such a high mortality rate, birth rates surely must have been high for man to have survived for so long. At the mercy of Nature's temperament, the worldwide population grew slowly over the centuries, eventually reaching a rough equilibrium at about ten million. Then, roughly 10,000 years ago, man changed Nature's ageless balance.

No one knows how or where, but humans discovered that the earth could be cultivated and brute animals, trained into submission. Wherever the agricultural revolution spread, it was quickly embraced. The arduous tasks of a hunting and

116

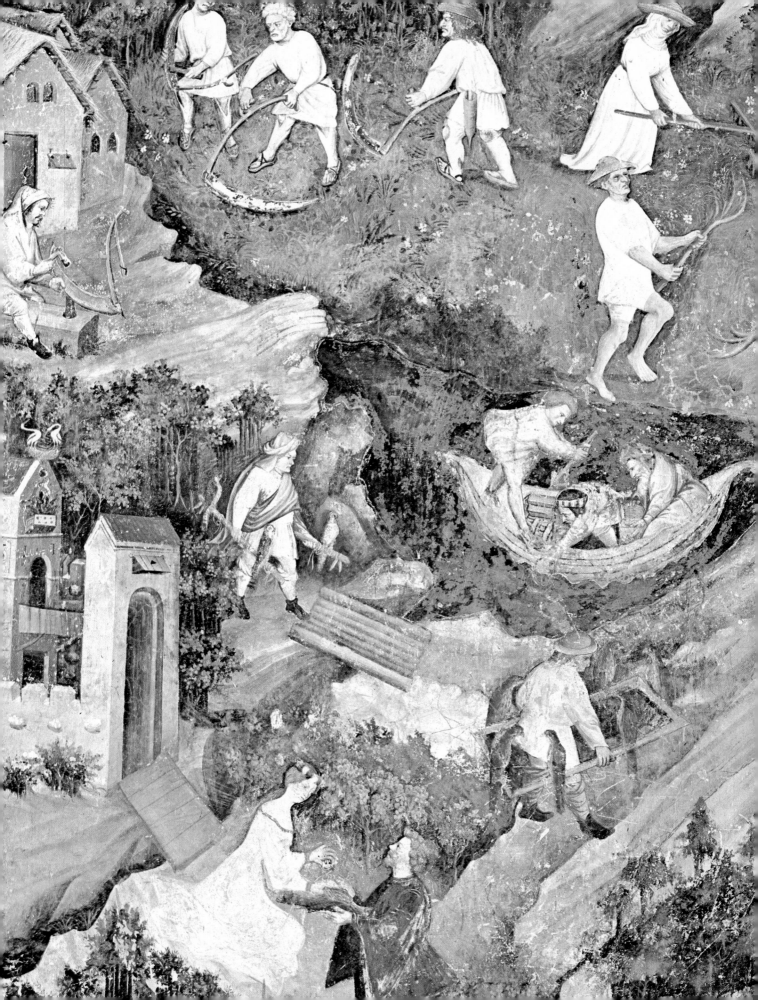

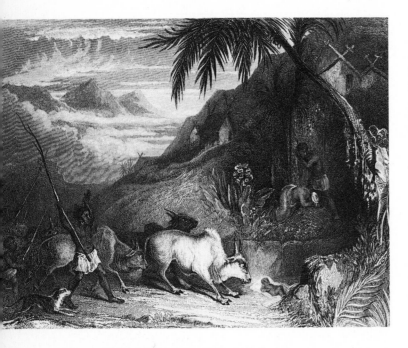

While Malagasy parents hide their eyes, cattle are driven over their infant, who had the misfortune to be born on an unlucky day. A product of superstition, convenience or harsh necessity, infanticide, in the view of nineteenth-century Irish historian William Lecky, was one of antiquity's "deepest stains."

gathering society were abandoned everywhere. Mobile camps settled into prototypes of the village. Early farmers labored over the earth and brought forth its bounty. Tools turned, making rough shelters more permanent. Metal-bladed plows and sturdier yokes broke tougher and tougher soil. Shoes for the horse and ox made them dependable farming machines. Man's inventiveness freed him from the ceaseless struggle to fill basic needs. Children became obvious economic benefits — more hands made lighter work. Population exploded.

By the birth of Christ, the ranks of humanity had increased thirtyfold to 300 million. The hunter-gatherer turned farmer-herdsman was a phenomenal success. With increasing numbers came the ever-increasing complexity of preserving order. The consequences of too many mouths to feed, the need to limit human numbers, were always deeply rooted in human awareness.

A Proper Population

Plato left it to the rulers of his utopian republic to determine "the size of the State and the proportionate amount of territory, beyond which they will not go." If the size of the state increased too quickly, unity would be lost. Sex should be regulated for eugenic reasons, thought Plato, to produce citizens suited to their regimented roles. He set the ideal population of a state at 5,040.

On these matters, the problem of diminishing food supplies seemed to influence Plato's pupil, Aristotle, more profoundly. Overpopulation bred poverty, the parent of revolution and crime. But Aristotle came to the same conclusion Plato had reached: a very populous city can rarely, if ever, be well governed. "All cities which have a reputation for good government," he said in *Politics*, "have a limit of population." He faulted Plato for not finding a mechanism by which population could be controlled, and in the same breath, promised to address the problem himself. He hardly kept the promise. Aristotle suggested that abortion might be the best method of population control. Perhaps unbeknownst to Aristotle, Plato did touch on another method of population control, infanticide, a common practice and a wickedly convenient holdover from harsher times.

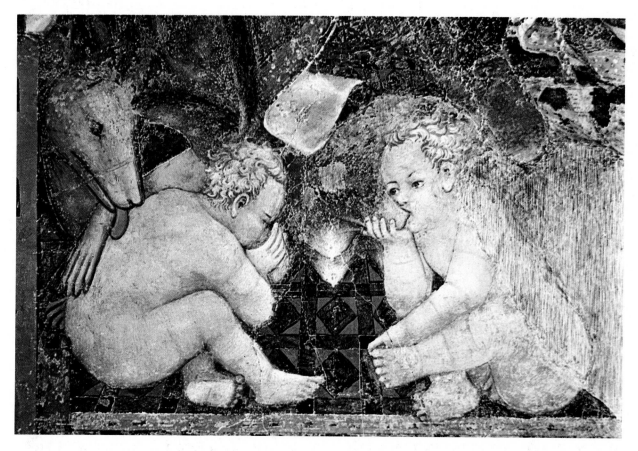

Because of the strict rules of inheritance and dowry customs, Hellenic Greek families were kept small. Usually, no more than one daughter was tolerated. Parents often drowned unwanted newborns or left them in the wilderness to die. The practice was adopted by Romans as a means to meet the pressures of life, either from economic necessity among the plebeians or an accepted convenience among patricians. Historian Edward Gibbon called infanticide the "stubborn vice of antiquity." It seems ironic that Rome's legendary founders, Romulus and Remus, abandoned by their parents on a hillside, were suckled rather than eaten by a she-wolf. History generally credits Christianity with the outlawing of infanticide in the fourth century A.D.

At the peak of Rome's glory, the dwindling birth rate so worried Augustus Caesar that he passed the *lex ludia de maritandis ordinibus.* The laws prohibited many restrictions on marriage and forbade the unmarried or childless of both sexes from receiving inheritances or legacies. Special privileges went to free women with three or more children, and divorces were curtailed by requiring at least seven witnesses. The laws caused immense resentment.

Rome's economy remained agricultural into imperial times. Her magnificent temples and constant warfare were more than moderate economic drains. The soil began to show signs of wear. Crowding encouraged epidemics. In the eastern Mediterranean, the population density had increased to roughly twenty-five individuals per square kilometer. In medieval times, population density in the region dropped to twenty and continued to fall. By the eighteenth century, it reached its lowest density, with ten people living in a square kilometer. With only the ox and plow to break ground, human population in many regions fluctuated around what seemed to be an

Thomas Robert Malthus

The Laws of Man's Multiplication

In the late winter of 1766, philosophers David Hume and Jean-Jacques Rousseau visited the English country mansion of their eccentric but devoted friend Daniel Malthus. Three weeks earlier, the Malthus family had grown by one, a boy, Thomas Robert, and each of the visitors — the mercurial Rousseau and the levelheaded Hume — gave the babe a kiss. The gesture, quipped one biographer, presumably assigned "diverse intellectual gifts" to the infant.

Thomas Robert Malthus grew into a tall, "elegantly formed" young man. Despite the speech impediment of a cleft palate, he became a preacher. As one of his admirers put it, "I would almost consent to speak as inarticulately, if I could think and act as wisely."

At the age of thirty-two, following a discussion with his father over the future of England's prosperity, he wrote an essay that would found the science of demography. *Essay on the Principle of Population* analyzed the growth of human numbers as a separate phenomenon, with dynamics and laws all its own. "Since the world began," he speculated, "the causes of population and depopulation have probably been as constant as any of the

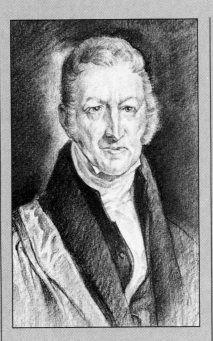

laws of nature with which we are acquainted."

What were the causes? Provided there is ample food, people will follow their passions and procreate. Human numbers increase faster than the earth's power to nourish them. When the gap widens, war, famine, pestilence and vice narrow it. Malthus's facts were not new. It was the inevitability he saw in the gloomy cycle that shocked the world.

An irritated Samuel Taylor Coleridge wrote in the margin of his copy of *On Population*, "Verbiage and senseless repetition. . . . Are we now to have a quarto to teach us that

great misery and great vice arise from poverty, and that there must be poverty in its worst shape wherever there are more mouths than loaves and more Heads than Brains?"

Malthus's diverse intellectual gifts led him further into the nascent science of economics. In 1805, at the age of thirty-nine, he was appointed to England's first chair of political economy, at the East India College in Haileybury. Using the pioneering tools of Adam Smith, Malthus greatly expanded the universe of economic thought with an intuition some called profound. "If only Malthus . . . had been the parent stem from which nineteenth-century economics proceeded," wrote British economist John Maynard Keynes in 1933, "what a much wiser and richer place the world would be today."

Malthus taught until his death in 1834. He had three children: a daughter who died in youth, another who married, and a son who died leaving behind no children.

Malthus's students called him "Pop." It can only be guessed if the nickname was an affectionate tribute to his scholastic guidance, a play on his clerical title or an inspired pun, abbreviating the subject he championed — population.

120

ecological limit. In a world of recurrent famine, plague and invasion, the idea of limiting the population would have seemed ludicrous. Despite sharp local fluctuations, however, mankind's overall numbers continued, slowly, to rise. In the eighteenth century, the negative implications of this steady growth earned a place among the vital issues confronting all humanity.

The Reverend's Theory

It began in eighteenth-century England with a friendly debate between Daniel Malthus, a land-owner, and his son Robert, a minister. Farming in Great Britain had become an enormously profit-able enterprise and Daniel was full of optimism. Population growth, as he saw it, encouraged eco-nomic growth. The more mouths there were to feed, the better it was for business. It was all in Adam Smith's *Inquiry into the Nature and Causes of the Wealth of Nations*, a work published in 1776 that laid the foundation for the science of politi-cal economy. But Robert Malthus had read the work in a different light and disagreed with his father. He studied the growth pattern and argued that it could not go on forever.

In *An Essay on the Principle of Population*, which he published in 1798, Malthus summed up his thoughts on the matter. The work hinges on two simple postulates: that food is necessary for man to exist and passion between the sexes is not only necessary but also permanent. Malthus went on to prove that the momentum of population growth was greater than the ability of the earth to sustain it. He applied Adam Smith's mathe-matics to the task. Farms increased in size arith-metically, that is, by addition. Fields could be added to fields, yields could increase steadily. But humanity increased geometrically. Man mul-tiplied. Like Plato before him, Malthus believed the happiness of a nation depended on how closely the growth rates could be matched.

The classic example of geometric growth is found in the legend of the man who invented chess. The king who commissioned the amuse-ment was so delighted that he invited the clever creator to name a reward. The inventor, more clever than the king realized, asked the king to place one grain of wheat on the first square of

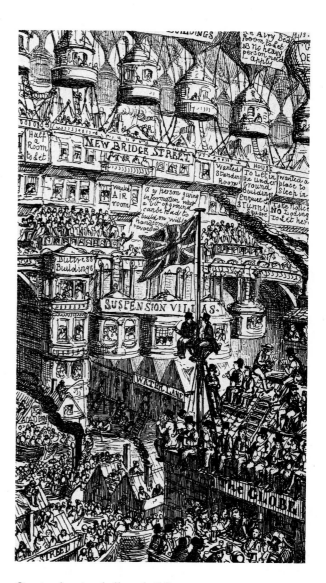

Streets of water, balloon buildings where heavy people need not apply, signs soliciting standing room all provide a backdrop for a busy day in Malthusian London. Nineteenth-century political satirist George Cruikshank mocked such alarmist views of population trends.

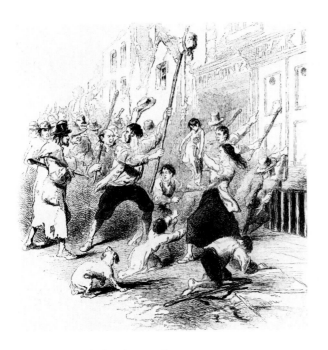

"For their food they have only potatoes and too few of them," wrote Sir Walter Scott in his Journal. *Aggravated by overpopulation, the 1845 failure of the potato crop resulted in the loss of two-and-a-half million lives. Food riots, such as the one pictured above from the 1846* Pictorial Times, *were common.*

the board, two on the second, four on the third, eight on the fourth, doubling the number of grains for each subsequent square. The king readily agreed, but fulfilling the promise proved impossible. By square twenty-one, the grains of wheat would reach a million. A billion would come only six squares later; and halfway, at square thirty-two, the figure would hit twenty-one billion. The pile of wheat necessary to fulfill the inventor's request has been estimated to be as much grain as the continent of North America has ever produced.

The Reverend Malthus realized that such a flood of humanity was unlikely. Under the "killing frost" of misery, fiery passions cooled. "Were every man sure of a comfortable provision for a family, almost every man would have one," he wrote. War, famine and pestilence were part of Nature's law and would always prune the unchecked growth of the human tree.

The theory's appeal lay in its simplicity. All England read it. Englishmen became Malthusians or anti-Malthusians. Many thought it a direct critique of the Poor Laws — an attempt to relieve the low wages and inflation brought on by the war with France in 1793. Subsidizing the poor only encouraged them to have larger families, taxpayers complained. "Bachelors and spinsters I decidedly venerate," pronounced Mr. Fax, the Malthus of satirical fiction. "The world is overstocked with featherless bipeds. More men than corn is a fearful pre-eminence." Others, more outraged, contended that Malthus was trying to blame the condition of the poor on their own indigence. "There is only one man too many on this earth," wrote French socialist Pierre-Joseph Proudhon, "and that is Mr. Malthus." Critics accused Malthus of presenting nothing more than a string of obvious conclusions masquerading as a theory, something that could never be proved or disproved. Fifty years later, however, the potato famine in Ireland brought to England's doorstep a demonstration of Nature's Malthusian methods, a display so graphic that England looked away.

The potato, a New World plant, had had its troubles in Ireland. There had been twenty-four crop failures by 1844. But on the whole, the potato flourished in Ireland's rocky soil and was the

Spindles whirling in a white flurry
shuttled the Industrial Revolution
into Georgia at the turn of the
century. Shattering the old ways,
technology came as a mixed blessing,
promising problems and progress.

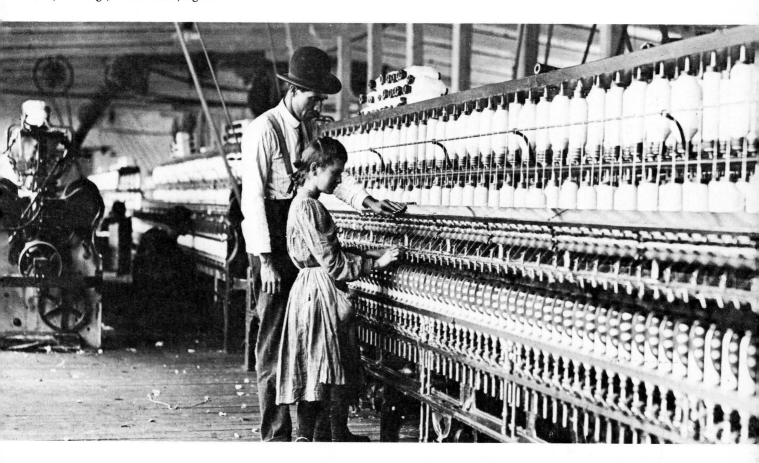

staple of the country. But the failure of 1845, complicated by humid weather more conducive to the growth of potato blight than potatoes, brought on famine. The lack of food was only aggravated by overpopulation. Waves of fever swept the island. By January 1847, coffins were "unprocurable." Funeral upon funeral, thousands of corpses abandoned along roads leading to ports of emigration, countless anonymous burials all burned into the Irish memory an image that would never be erased. Nearly a third of the population was lost. By the turn of the century there were more Irishmen in North America than in Ireland. Those who stayed behind accused the English of not doing enough, of being cold-hearted monsters who invoked Malthusian explanations to justify the lack of help. The enmity sown during the famine persisted.

The means to free man from so direct a dependency on unpredictable farming techniques were already being developed. Technology catapulted mankind into an unprecedented relationship with Nature. It began with Englishman James Watt's steam engine, which went into commercial use in the 1780s. By 1850, steam was providing the power of four million horses worldwide. Energy led to new energy. In 1859, American Edwin Drake proved he could bring crude oil to the earth's surface by drilling. The next year, 600 oil companies were incorporated in Pennsylvania alone, and French engineer J. E. Lenoir was awarded a patent for a gas engine. Electrical generators were widely available a decade later.

The Industrial Revolution flourished hand in hand with a "mortality revolution," brought on by medical advances. Better farming led to better nutrition and thus better resistance to disease. Soap and sounder housing cut down on diseases associated with crowding. Cotton underwear replaced wool, reducing diseases spread by lice.

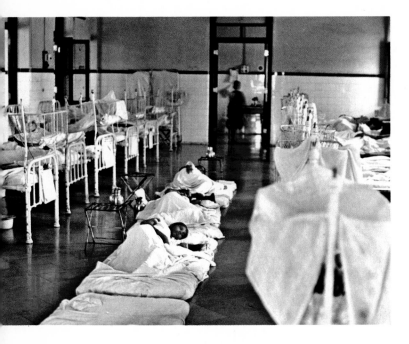

This crowded maternity ward in Bombay, India, is a poignant reminder of the country's chronic population pressures. India's population is larger than that of North and Latin America combined.

Sanitation helped purge plague and cholera. By the late 1940s, vaccinations had dramatically cut the death toll from typhoid fever, tuberculosis, diphtheria and other diseases. Malaria fell to the onslaught of DDT. The scale balancing births and deaths tilted again. Technology's benefits were reflected in human numbers.

Where it had taken mankind several million years to reach its first billion in 1800, it took only the next 130 years to reach its second billion. The third billion arrived only 30 years later in 1960, and the fourth, a mere 15 years after that. Before the end of this century the human population could reach six billion — roughly a tenth of all the people who have ever lived could be on hand to welcome the twenty-first century. It has been predicted that if this pattern of growth continues, there will be, by the twenty-sixth century, one human being for every square yard of dry land on the earth. Confronted with such a prediction, Malthusian logic leads to ominous conclusions. Something will happen to limit human numbers long before they grow so large. We can predict the fact, but not the means.

The Industrial Revolution divided the world into developed nations, who have mastered and most directly benefited from technology, and developing nations, who still depend on agriculture and are trying to foment their own industrial revolutions. The "mortality revolution" came in stages in developed countries. Between 1700 and 1900, even though the population in industrialized countries grew two to three times faster than the rest of the world, birth rates came down gradually. In a humanitarian fervor, the medical advances of the mortality revolution were exported to developing countries all at once, with what economist Carlo Cipolla calls "appalling consequences." The drop in death rate that had occurred in Europe over most of two centuries happened in developing countries in a matter of decades. Now developing countries are growing more than twice as fast as developed ones. Snared in a vicious Malthusian trap, these countries look to a second wave of the industrial revolution as their great hope. "All that 'exploding' underdeveloped countries need," writes Cipolla, "is to bring down their birth rates to a manageable level." To blame all of the Third World's woes on overpopulation is to oversimplify. But most experts agree that fewer deaths must be balanced by fewer births, and some see population growth as the poisoned soil out of which the other miseries of underdevelopment grow.

But with a commitment to lower birth rates, the problem shifts from the global, humanitarian concerns of unimaginable numbers and an uncertain future to the most intimate and personal decisions of human experience. National policies and demographic arguments have trouble forcing their way into the bedroom. But people have long been in the business of controlling the size of families. An enormous variety of potions and tricks, hybrids of magic and tried technique, express a universal desire for a practical, effective contraceptive, an alternative to abstinence, abortion and infanticide.

Piripiri and Other Potions

The Ait Sadden of Morocco once believed that if a man ate the knotted and boiled oviduct of a hen, his partner would incur a permanent curse of sterility. Natives of the Oasis of Sima in Libya would inscribe a formula from the Koran on a parchment and then sew the parchment into a pouch, which they wore around their waists during coitus to avoid pregnancy. They were also said to enhance this method's effectiveness by anointing the genitals with foam from a camel's mouth. Medicine men of the Cherokee Indians generally kept their secrets well guarded, but anthropologist Frans Olbrecht found an informant among them. Cherokee women believed they could induce sterility by eating roots of the spotted cowbane, known as "beaver poison," for four successive days. If a Canelos woman of South America drank piripiri tea, followed by a strict diet of unsalted, roasted plantain and small forest fowl, tribal custom said she could live with a man without becoming pregnant. Potions and charms to prevent pregnancy appear worldwide, but of more interest to modern science are techniques, ancient and modern, grounded in physiological realities.

Egyptian papyri prescribe several alternative methods of contraception, which, at first glance, appear to be more the products of superstition than of the generally sophisticated medical knowledge Egyptian physicians had gained. Modern investigations suggest that not only were the ancient techniques more than charms, they also prefigured present-day methods. A pessary, or intravaginal barrier, made of pulverized crocodile dung and paste might have effectively blocked the passage of sperm into the uterus. As well as being a physical barrier, the alkaline dung probably upset the precise acid-base balance in the vagina that allows sperm to swim to their target. Another prescribed device, a lint tampon soaked in extract of acacia tips, must have also been an effective contraceptive. The acacia extract, lactic acid, is a commonly used spermicide today. The ancient technique of coating the vagina with honey, natron or other oily or gummy substances is the basis for many contraceptive suppositories now used.

Anthropologist Margaret Mead found that the Samoans practiced coitus interruptus, the withdrawal by the male before ejaculation. According to her analysis, the practice was not the consequence of exposure to the ways of the white man. The Nandi of East Africa today practice a rustic rhythm method, warning young girls not

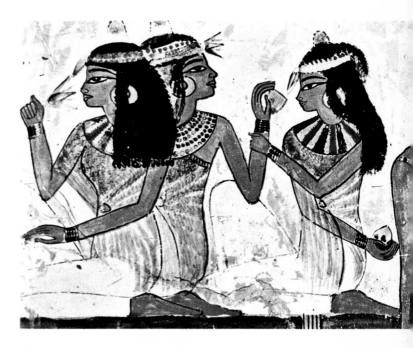

Egyptian women at a banquet pass the mandragora, or mandrake, root. Their feast is immortalized in a 3,500-year-old fresco on the tomb of Prince Nakht. Ascribed magical powers through the ages, the root, which is shaped like a human body, was both fertility drug and contraceptive to the ancient Egyptians. Today, podophyllum, a derivative of mandragora, is used to treat warts and moles.

125

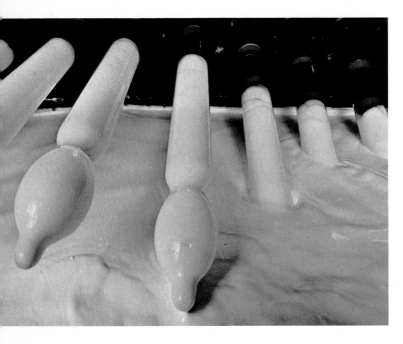

Emerging from the dipping stage of production, condom molds move along a conveyer belt. Each mold is coated with a thin film of synthetic rubber that will dry into a condom, a popular birth control device.

to visit the warriors' huts for a specified number of days after menstruation. Coitus interruptus is also known to their neighbors, the Maasai. The black women of Martinique and Guiana have long used douches of lemon juice and extract from the husks of the mahogany nut. Modern analysis has demonstrated that one or two tablespoons of lemon juice in a quart of water makes a citric acid solution strong enough to immobilize sperm immediately.

Casanova's Legacy

The idea of covering the penis also dates back to antiquity. The ancient Egyptians and Romans wore decorative silk sheaths and animal bladders more for protection against venereal disease than to prevent pregnancy. Sixteenth-century Italian anatomist Gabriello Fallopio developed a modest cap of linen to cover only the head of the penis. The sheaths became popular with libertines, most notable of whom was eighteenth-century Italian adventurer Casanova, who called them "Redingotes d'Angleterre," or English riding coats — "the overcoat that puts one's mind at rest." Casanova is generally credited with promoting the contraceptive qualities of the sheath. Scottish biographer and rake James Boswell more than once mentioned his "armour." The origin of the word "condom" is enigmatic. It suddenly appeared in England in the eighteenth century and spread with the device's popularity. One rumor has it that a modest pharmacist lent his name to the brand he sold, then changed his name and disavowed his invention.

With the vulcanization of rubber in the mid-nineteenth century, the use of condoms skyrocketed. The London Rubber Company, which began in the back room of a tobacco shop in 1916, was, by 1960, marketing over two-and-a-half million condoms a week. The condom has many advantages: not only is it safe, readily available and inexpensive, it also inhibits the transmission of venereal disease and gives the man a role in birth control.

In the 1830s, Wilhelm Mensinga, a German physician, popularized another rubber contraceptive shield, invented by his countryman Friedrich Adolph Wilde. Working on the same principle as the condom, it fits inside the woman, blocking sperm from entering the cervix. The shield became popular in Holland, and by the time it reached England it wore the name "Dutch cap." The cap evolved into what is now one of the most popular birth control devices — the diaphragm. A flexible rubber dome, the diaphragm fits against the vaginal walls, covering the cervix and holding a small quantity of spermicide. Tests have shown that when used correctly it fails only about 2 percent of the time.

Available in England, the cervical cap is a variation of the diaphragm that the U. S. Food and Drug Administration has not approved and therefore has not been distributed in the United States. The thimble-shaped rubber dome fits onto the cervix and holds a dosage of spermicide against the tissue. Some American researchers are wary of the device. They worry that the pinch of the cap might damage the cervix.

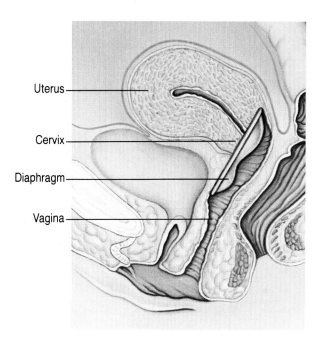

Lippes Loops and Birnberg Bows

Anyone visiting a certain medical conference in New York City in 1964 might have been intrigued to find doctors from all over the world arguing about Lippes loops, Birnberg bows and Marguilies spirals. Plastic coils and figure eights, wheels with tails and nylon rings bore these and other names. All of them were cheap, costing only pennies to make, but these odd devices were to stir up a heated controversy that is yet to be resolved. Fitted not over the cervix but inside the uterus itself, these tiny tools prevented pregnancy. But were they safe?

Farmers and ranchers have known for centuries that inserting metal objects into the uteruses of livestock discouraged pregnancy. None knew why. After World War I, German physician Ernst Gräfenberg began implanting gold and silver rings in the uteruses of hundreds of women. His results encouraged other doctors to try similar techniques, but their devices did not work well. Women bled, fetuses were aborted, and the practice was abandoned. In 1959, two studies, one in Israel and the other in Japan, resurrected the idea. Today, some sixty million women worldwide use intrauterine devices, or IUDs. The devices prevent pregnancy more than 90 percent of the time.

Researchers suspect that the presence of any foreign object in the womb inhibits the implantation of a fertilized egg by inflaming the wall of the uterus. Some scientists think an IUD may also dislodge a fertilized egg that has been implanted on the uterine wall. Others speculate that the IUD could somehow allow the ovum to descend from the Fallopian tube too quickly to be fertilized. Still others believe that the device might also impale sperm, preventing them from traveling to the Fallopian tubes.

American birth control clinics currently shy away from prescribing IUDs. A main reason is discomfort. For six weeks after fitting, the uterus will try to expel the device, causing painful cramps. There is also a high incidence of inflammatory pelvic disease, especially among users of the IUD who have more than one sex partner. More troubling, the presence of the device somehow allows pelvic infection to spread into the Fallopian tubes. These fragile passageways are easily scarred, collapsed or sealed, and high infertility rates are often associated with IUDs. The devices can also cause scarring or damage to the uterine wall, the consequences of which may not show up until pregnancy, threatening the development of the fetus. An ideal candidate for an

127

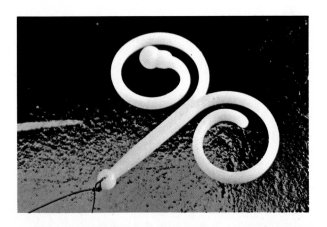

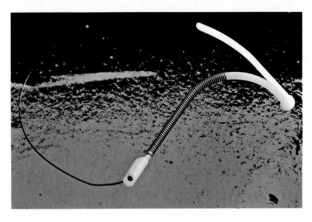

Two of the most widely used intrauterine devices, the Saf-T-Coil, *top, and the* Copper-7, *look almost like toys or gadgets. Fitted in the uterus, the IUD is an effective birth control device.*

IUD might be a woman who already has a family, only one partner, light menstrual periods and no abnormal Pap smears.

The inconvenience and side effects of many contraceptive methods have kept alive the search for an effective oral contraceptive. A long sought goal of contraceptive technology has been some brew or substance more reliable than the mandrake, wormwood and edderwort prescribed by first-century Greek physician Dioscorides. An effective contraceptive pill appeared on the market in the 1960s, but only after much exploration of the biochemistry of menstruation and ovulation, and the work of two remarkable people.

In 1912, Margaret Sanger was posted as a visiting nurse in New York City's East Side, a sweltering, crowded ghetto. She was appalled by the conditions brought on by the crowding, the all too frequent five-dollar back-room abortions, and worse, the ignorance. Immigrant women begged her to tell them how the rich managed to limit the size of their families. There was no special secret, she told them, nothing mysterious about condoms or withdrawal. Whether or not the women of New York's East Side were satisfied with her answer, Sanger herself was not. She began to publish *Woman Rebel*, a feminist magazine urging women to "look the whole world in the face with a go-to-hell look" and to stand up for the rights "to be lazy, to be an unmarried mother, to destroy, to create, to love, [and] live." But it was a small pamphlet, *Family Limitation*, that caused the loudest uproar. By explicitly describing methods of contraception, the pamphlet violated nine federal statutes. Over the next decades, Sanger was jailed eight times. But in the name of Malthus and feminism, she fought to found the birth control movement in America.

Sanger's relentless promotion of birth control led to a chance meeting in 1950 with Gregory Pincus, Director of the Worcester Foundation for Experimental Biology. Their discussion was private and never recorded, but Sanger apparently complained of the unreliability of contraceptive methods available at the time. She evidently asked Pincus, who was familiar with the chemistry of ovulation in laboratory animals, why it was not possible to chemically limit fertility.

Margaret Sanger

A Revolutionary's Lonely Vision

On a sweltering mid-July night in 1912, Jake Sachs, a truck driver, arrived home at his little flat on New York City's Lower East Side to find his children huddled around their mother on the living room floor. She had tried to give herself an abortion and was near death from blood poisoning. Sachs called a doctor, who in turn called a young nurse named Margaret Sanger. The two-week ordeal to save the woman's life began just as a vicious heat wave hit the city. Sanger stayed at her patient's bedside. The neighbors brought ice and groceries.

When Sadie Sachs finally recovered she seemed more frightened than grateful. "Another child will finish me, I suppose?" she asked the nurse, who looked to the doctor for an answer. He admonished her that any further foolishness would make another visit by him unnecessary. After brooding, the patient finally blurted out: "But how can I prevent it?" The physician chuckled awkwardly and made evasive jokes as he left. "You want to have your cake and eat it, too," he said. "Tell Jake to sleep on the roof." Sanger, silent in the doctor's presence, watched a shadow of despondency pass over the patient's face. Three

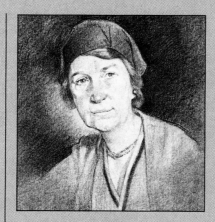

months later Sadie Sachs was dead from the same brutal surgery, this time at the hands of a back-room abortionist. Sanger arrived at her bedside in time to watch her die.

Till three in the morning, the frail young nurse wandered in a daze through the streets of New York, oblivious to the heavy nurse's bag she carried. Later the same morning, looking through her window down onto the hushed streets, she envisioned with stark clarity "women writhing in travail to bring forth little babies; the babies themselves naked and hungry, wrapped in newspapers to keep them from the cold; six-year-old children with pinched, pale, wrinkled faces, old in concentrated wretchedness, pushed into gray and fetid cellars, crouching on stone floors." She would never be the same

again. She closed her mind and heart to all other causes and gave herself to one goal — the birth control movement in America was born.

Denounced by doctors, censured by churches, ridiculed in the press, abandoned by even her most liberal friends, she fought almost alone, challenging the Comstock censorship laws to bring contraception information to all women. She was jailed eight times. Even her father, an impetuously outspoken Irishman, grew impatient with her cause. "Margaret, can't you find some other subject in the world to talk about besides the bedroom?" he asked, whispering the word bedroom. But Margaret, an avowed educator and agitator, was fond of the saying, "There is nothing as powerful as an idea whose time has come."

Sanger saw her fight as the fight for life. Through the years of struggle, she felt that the most momentous human experience was witnessing the birth of a child. The visionary Victorian author, H. G. Wells, called her the greatest woman in the world. He predicted that by allowing men and women to control their own destinies, the work she had begun would become the most influential in mankind's history.

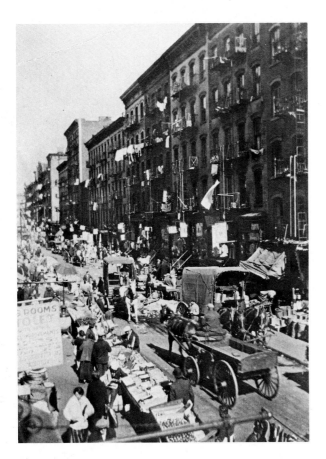

Cradle of the American birth control movement, the Brownsville section of New York City was the site of Margaret Sanger's first clinic. The clinic's sign at 46 Amboy Street may have been hard to find. But it did not escape the notice of police, who immediately closed the clinic and jailed Sanger.

Since the 1920s, scientists had gradually been unraveling the role of hormones in sexual stimulation, ovulation and pregnancy. Pincus thought the best means of preventing conception might lie in manipulating these hormones and limiting ovulation — with no egg, there could be no fertilization. He knew that once an egg is fertilized, a woman does not continue to ovulate because of the presence of progesterone in her blood. He also knew that progesterone postpones the regular menstrual cycle for the nine months of pregnancy. The problem, Pincus decided, was in finding an abundant source of the chemical. Tons of processed mammal ovaries from slaughterhouses yielded only hundredths of an ounce. But hormones similar to progesterone had been found in relative abundance in certain plants, so the search focused on the plant kingdom.

There are at least a quarter of a million species of flowering plants in the world. About 630 of these are known as Dioscoreaceae, named for the Greek physician who had exhaustively catalogued the contraceptive properties of hundreds of herbs. Mostly tropical climbers, the plants appear on six of the seven continents. Their most widely known representative is the yam. The flowers are small, regular and inconspicuous in the lush jungles where they grow wild. In the tropics of Veracruz Mexico, a wild yam known to the Mexicans as *cabeza de negro,* "the black-headed one," proved, after a long search, to be a rich source of the material necessary to produce progesterone on a large scale. Pincus established the principle that would lead to the first effective oral contraceptive.

The pill caught on. After a decade on the market, an estimated ten million women around the world were using it. An early controversy arose in England over the pill's safe use. A group called the Genetic Study Unit began looking into the pill's possible side effects. The *London Sunday Times* discovered, however, that the group had strong attachments to the giant London Rubber Company, producer of condoms.

Further research and reports from physicians around the world have revealed that the pill is not without serious side effects. The list of reported symptoms is sobering. The pill can cause nausea, weight gain, fatigue, depression, loss of sex drive, increase in breast size and tenderness, dilated veins in the legs and other complications. Together, physician and woman can avoid most of these problems by shifting the proportion of hormones in the dosage. But the long-term effects of the pill remain a nagging question.

Scientists know the pill works, but as with the IUD, they don't know exactly how. The pill may work by a combination of mechanisms. One explanation holds that the hormones in the pill change the womb's internal environment to prevent the implantation of a fertilized egg. Another suggests that it also alters the composition of the natural shield of mucus that guards the cervix, either killing sperm or prohibiting them from penetrating the uterus. The most widely accepted explanation is that the artificially introduced hormones disrupt the chain of hormonal messages that releases an egg once a month.

Unhappy with the need for daily doses and convinced that the pill worked by a combination of mechanisms, M. C. Chang, one of Pincus's fellow researchers, experimented with hormones administered to animals once they mated. He found that strong doses of norethynodrel (the main ingredient of Pincus's original pill) prevented pregnancy. While no "morning-after" pill has been approved for general use by the U. S. Food and Drug Administration, an effective contraceptive after intercourse is available to victims of rape and incest. A morning-after prescription is nothing more than four ordinary birth control pills taken at one time.

Another method of administering birth control hormones is the Depo-Provera shot. Injecting this form of progesterone directly into muscle tissue effectively suppresses the luteinizing hormone necessary for ovulation. Lasting three months, it is a good contraceptive for women who, for various reasons, cannot accept the responsibility of daily birth control measures or who do not want the side effects. A serious drawback to Depo-Provera is a warning. The physician must tell the woman "she may not be able to become pregnant" after taking the drug.

In the 1970s, a five-year study involving more than 800 women in Brazil, Chile, Denmark and

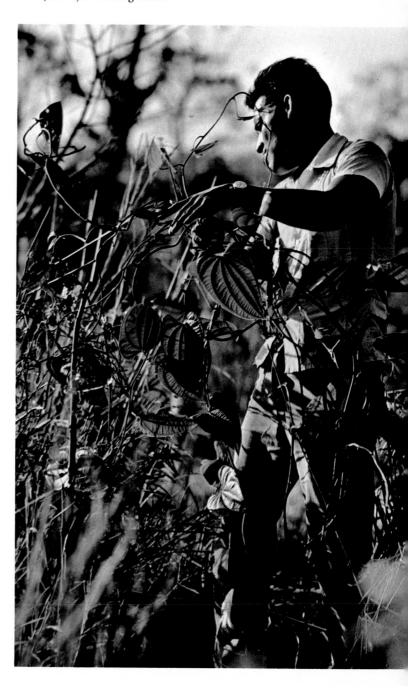

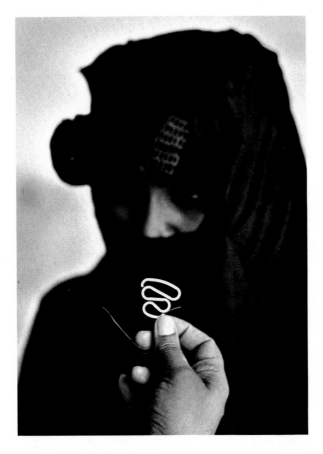

Finland tested the effectiveness of timed-release contraceptive capsules. In a single operation, six capsules were implanted in the skin of the forearm. The biodegradable shells of the capsules broke down in sequence, preventing pregnancy for five years. For the 640 women who did not withdraw from the experiment, the method proved 99 percent effective.

Even advanced methods of birth control may not succeed in solving the problem of overpopulation. "Shocking as it may seem," wrote professor S. Chandrasekhar of the University of California in 1961, "in many rural areas the cost of having a baby would be cheaper than the price of birth control equipment." His belief abruptly tempers optimism for advances in contraceptive technology and their potential for solving chronic population problems. He was speaking of India in particular, a country plagued by the number of its people. Measuring only 2.4 percent of the earth's total land area, India holds 15 percent of the world's population. When India gained independence from Great Britain in 1947, its population was about 344 million. Since then the figure has doubled and is still rising.

A Subcontinent's Struggles

An ambitious family planning program had been under way in India since the early 1950s. Because more than three-fourths of India's people still live in some 600,000 rural villages, family planning workers had not only to travel to all of these villages, but also persuade the villagers that India's future depended on their controlling the number of new births. In these villages, children have always been considered an economic asset. Each new mouth to feed comes with a pair of hands that can be put to work in the fields. The villagers argued that they needed large families to survive. With 30 percent of all children dying before the age of five, families wanted to have as many children as possible. Many of the family planning workers carrying contraceptives and birth control information to the villages were urban, poorly trained and ill-equipped to meet these arguments. Moslems and Hindus alike abhorred the idea of abortion and resisted the pill, condom and IUD.

In a desperate attempt to overcome such obstacles, the government initiated a sterilization campaign in the mid-1970s. Brightly colored tents, posters and flags appeared throughout the countryside. With all the trappings of a carnival, loudspeakers blared out the new patriotism: Do your national duty! Be sterilized! But when these public relations techniques failed, the government resorted to coercion. With no official declarations and no legislation, India enforced family planning with a nightmarish ferocity. A sinister certificate of sterilization became the equivalent of papers of citizenship. Without one, people were barred from hospitals, unless they consented to sterilization during the visit. Minor officials withheld housing, food-rationing tickets and driver's licenses. A bank clerk told one woman that she could make no withdrawals from her savings account unless she produced proof of sterilization. Villagers hid in the fields from ster-

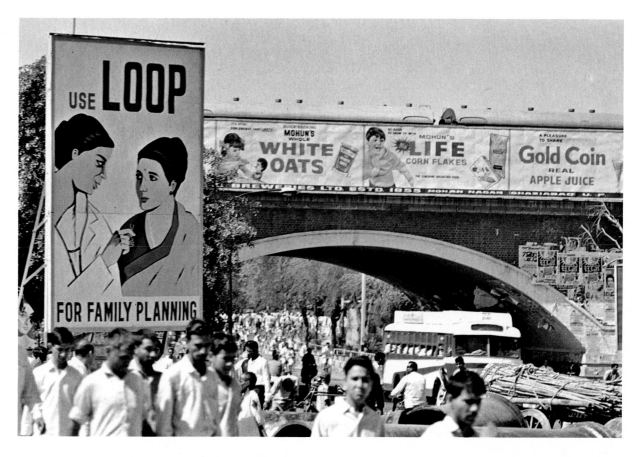

ilization squads. The government tried to ban press coverage, but the prestigious Bombay journal, the *Fulcrum,* reported an incident in the small town of Barsi. Determined to meet the weekly quota of 1,000 sterilizations, the police abducted several hundred men, threw them into garbage trucks and drove them to family planning clinics. At the clinics, police held the men down while vasectomies were performed. Among those abducted was Shahu Laxman Ghalake, a poor peasant who was visiting Barsi that day. He was beaten and kicked, and when he tried to explain that he had been sterilized at least ten years earlier, the police and workers at the clinic ignored him. Three men held him down while another tried to sterilize him again.

In September 1976, the Indian government passed a law stating that as of January 1977, all government workers would undergo sterilization after their third child or lose their jobs. Indira Gandhi was voted out of office in March 1977. The campaign had nearly doubled its goal of 4.3 million sterilizations, reaching 7.8 million by early 1977. Despite the drastic measures, the growth rate of India's population during the 1970s was only .05 percent lower than in the 1960s.

According to the Population Reference Bureau, more than thirty developing countries have shown 20 to 60 percent decreases in birth rates over the past decade. Birth rates also tend to fall with economic well-being, which many experts see as another hopeful trend. Development in the world's poor nations is coming to be seen by many as the best contraceptive.

The worldwide distribution of effective but still mysterious contraceptives has been called the largest uncontrolled experiment in history. Can the human fabric be tailored to fit the earth, or have we tampered irreversibly with a balance more fragile than we ever realized?

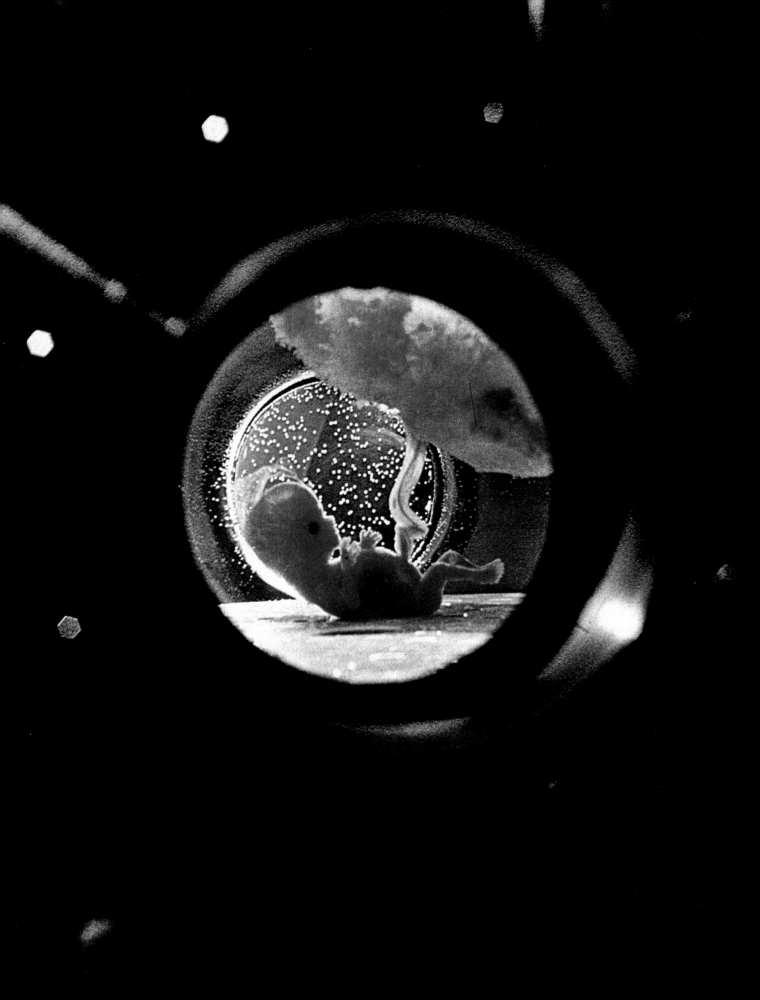

Chapter 6

Braving the New World

Through the creations of science, mankind can now control or influence events that were never before within the realm of choice. Once feared diseases have been banished, boundaries of distance, climate and terrain have been erased. With a mixture of excitement and apprehension, we are moving swiftly into an unfamiliar future that seems more perplexing the more we ponder it. Reproduction, formerly thought to be in the hands only of Nature or God, has now yielded to man's touch. Although growth in population runs on unabated in many parts of the world, it has been slowed elsewhere by the intervention of birth control.

Apart from the consequences of overpopulation, quite another problem brings anguish into the lives of many people. Roughly ten million American men and women are infertile for one reason or another, and the number is rising. About three-and-a-half million married couples in the United States — one in every six — cannot have children. For many, the burden of being childless becomes a painful disappointment. Infertility is a problem that has persisted through the ages. George Washington, the father of his country, fathered no children of his own.

Under the best of circumstances, it is not always easy to bring a child into the world. A woman's chances of becoming pregnant in any given month are generally between 10 and 20 percent, although in teen-agers the possibility is at least twice as great. It takes the average couple about six months before they can conceive a child. Most often, the cause of infertility lies with a hormonal or physical deficiency in one partner, but social trends and changes in the environment can also play a part. Although the peak of fertility is between the ages of eighteen and twenty, more women are waiting until they are well into their thirties to have children. As more and more women take to strenuous exercise

The womb is indeed a "fine and private place," even when it is outside the mother's body. Here, a fetus lies in an artificial womb, a steel chamber filled with a solution similar to natural amniotic fluid. Many new medical advances have extended the hope of life as science probes the wonders of birth.

for fitness, they can unwittingly lower their ability to reproduce. For women who run more than ten miles a week, the exercise can be too much of a good thing. They are much more likely than other women to stop ovulating entirely. When they give up running, they frequently become fertile once again. As women age, they naturally get heavier. The desire to be fashionably thin, however, carries a risk of infertility. Trying to maintain a youthful weight often upsets a woman's hormonal system, causing her to be infertile. If she adds a few pounds, she can usually recover her fertility.

Studies of infertility in men have revealed that the most important factor is not so much the number of sperm cells a man has but their motility, or ability to move and enter the egg. The average number of sperm cells is about 60 million per cubic centimeter, but a man can be normally fertile with a concentration ranging anywhere between 5 million and 120 million.

Doctors are finding that infertility once ascribed to psychological problems frequently has direct physical causes. Complications of surgery or disease in the pelvic region may also produce infertility or impotence. Some neurological problems or disorders affecting metabolism or blood flow can make men infertile, as well. Another cause of infertility in men is the varicocele, a condition marked by varicose veins in the testicles. About 15 percent of all men have the condition, but most suffer no loss of fertility from it. Blood pools inside the dilated veins and interferes with the production of normal sperm cells by raising the internal temperature of the testicles. With a simple operation, doctors can tie off a faulty vein that allows blood to lag in the testicles. Healthy vessels can then carry blood back to the abdomen. Between 20 and 40 percent of the patients who undergo the operation show a dramatic rise in sperm count.

Childbirth's Chances

Infertility is an anxiety for an increasing number of women. Although women are born with about 600,000 eggs in their ovaries, as much as two-thirds of all infertility is the result of defective ovulation. Normally, one egg matures every

month and is released from an ovary when it is ripe for fertilization. In some cases, though, the ovary may not release the egg at the right time, meaning that it cannot become fertilized because it is too young or past maturity. On occasion, the ovaries do not relinquish any eggs at all or will do so only infrequently.

Besides these physical limitations, the stress of modern living can affect fertility. In the United States and other developed countries, women have pursued careers in unprecedented numbers in recent years. Such women frequently postpone childbearing until they are beyond the age of thirty. A 1982 study of French women indicates that fertility declines after age thirty and falls even more sharply after thirty-five. Whether women who want to have children should change their goals somewhat and seek to start their families before settling into careers has become a matter of some controversy.

Another modern convention, contraception, has been known to render women sterile or temporarily infertile. Infections from intrauterine devices have curtailed some women's reproductive capacity, birth control pills have stopped ovulation in some women and abortions have left behind infections or scars that make pregnancy difficult. Venereal disease can also damage the reproductive tract.

A common cause of female infertility, affecting as much as a third of all barren women, is blocked Fallopian tubes, or oviducts, as they are also called. Without healthy Fallopian tubes, the egg, even if fertilized, can never reach the uterus to be implanted. Sometimes the oviducts do not develop properly or they become damaged by disease or injury. Modern surgical techniques have now made it possible for many once sterile women to bear children. Working under a microscope, surgeons can often repair the delicate walls of the Fallopian tubes, reopening a conduit for the egg. Someday it may be possible to transplant human Fallopian tubes, a feat surgeons have already accomplished in animals.

Disorders affecting the secretion of hormones often prevent normal ovulation and, on occasion, the maintenance of a pregnancy once it has occurred. Treatment with hormones similar to the

J. Marion Sims

The Gentleman Doctor

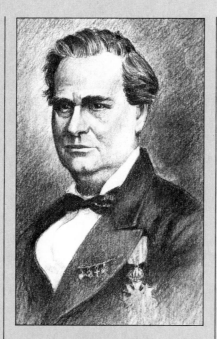

"If there was anything I hated," an early nineteenth-century physician once said, "it was investigating the organs of the female pelvis." The physician, J. Marion Sims, would later change his mind. Indeed, he achieved international recognition as a pioneer of gynecologic surgery and founder of gynecology as a medical specialty. His comment was notable for more than its irony, however, for it reflected the attitudes of not just one man but an entire profession.

The eldest of eight children born to a poor family, Sims was the only child his parents could afford to educate. His mother wanted him to become a minister; his father, a lawyer. Instead, Sims chose medicine, a profession his father viewed with contempt. "To think that *my* son should be going around from house to house through this country . . . to ameliorate human suffering," his father moaned, "is a thought I never supposed I should have to contemplate."

After graduating from medical school in 1835, Sims opened his own practice in Lancaster, South Carolina. But the venture spurred feelings of incompetence rather than pride. "I had had no clinical advantages, no hospital experience,

and had seen nothing at all of sickness," Sims recalled. When his first two patients, both infants, died, he hastily left town. He moved to Mt. Meigs, Alabama, where he bought another doctor's practice for $200. Here, finally, his success and reputation grew.

Ten years later, an accident sent his career in a fruitful new direction. The victim, a Mrs. Merrill, was thrown from a horse and suffered a painfully shifted uterus. Sims discovered he could examine her injury far easier when she raised her knees to her chest.

It was then that Sims had an inspired idea. A little earlier,

he had examined three women, all suffering from a vesico-vaginal fistula, a tear between the bladder and vagina resulting from childbirth. He had dismissed all three cases as incurable. Suddenly, he wondered whether that was true. He called one of the patients back and asked her to assume the same position Mrs. Merrill had. He could now see the injury clearly and was convinced it could be repaired.

His work was not immediately fruitful. It took many attempts before he found an appropriate suturing material, but eventually he met with success. Repeated many times over, the operation won Sims international fame.

He expanded the field he had begun by establishing America's first hospital for women in New York in 1855. And he crossed into new territory by experimenting in artificial insemination. His lone success in fifty-five attempts with various patients was one of the earliest ever, although the patient later miscarried.

Behind Sims's relentless energy was an enduring romanticism. He sought to ease the suffering of women, whom he called, in the manner of a quintessential Southern gentleman, "the loveliest of all God's creatures."

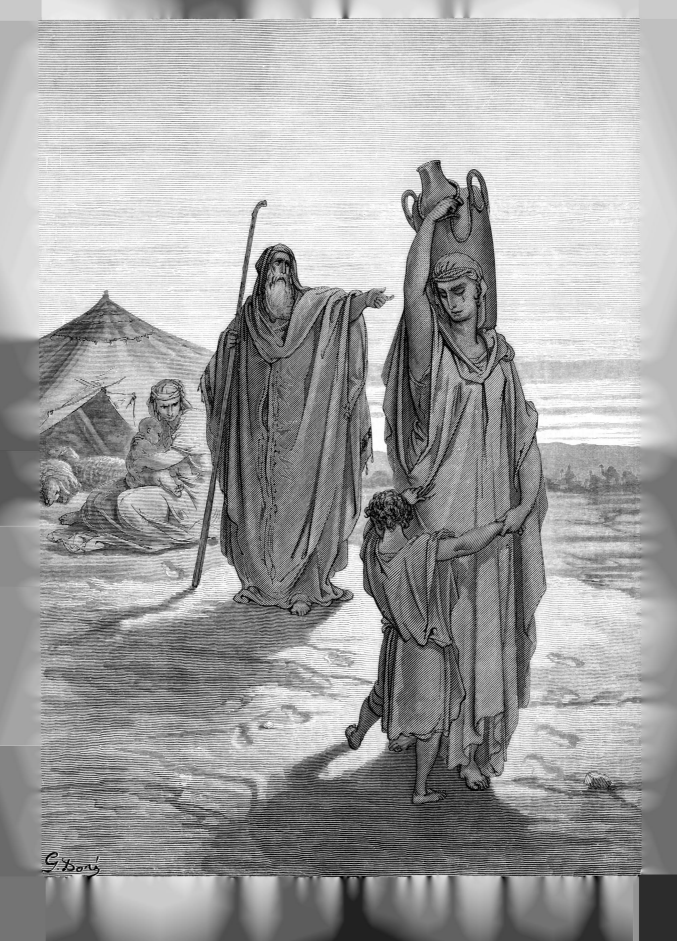

In the book of Genesis, Abraham banishes Hagar to appease his wife, Sarah. Hagar had borne him a son, Ishmael, because Sarah was barren. Outcasts to their masters, Hagar and Ishmael were blessed by God.

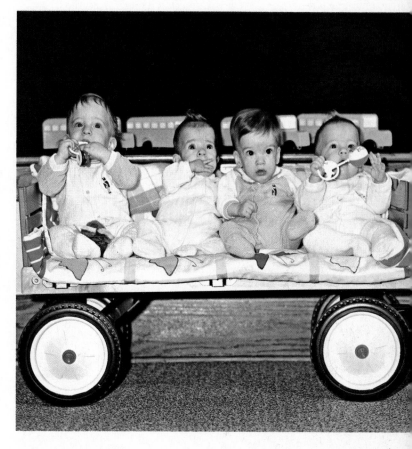

Born quintuplets, one of whom died, the Granata children of Toledo, Ohio are healthy, active infants. After their mother took a fertility drug to induce ovulation, several eggs matured simultaneously.

female hormone estrogen can stimulate ovulation. One such drug, Clomid, scientifically known as clomiphene citrate, induces ovulation in roughly 70 percent of the women who take it. About two-thirds of these women will later conceive. If Clomid fails to bring on ovulation, doctors can prescribe stronger hormones, the most common of which is human menopausal gonadotropin, also called Pergonal. Extracted from the urine of postmenopausal women, the drug induces ovulation in about 90 percent of the women taking it, with pregnancy following for two-thirds of those women. Pergonal is a powerful fertility drug that can stimulate the maturation and release of more than one egg at a time. In 1981, a woman who had taken Pergonal gave birth to quintuplets in Toledo, Ohio. Other hormones not yet in wide use may induce pregnancy by acting on the pituitary gland, the "master gland" governing hormonal secretions from other endocrine glands.

Female infertility is not simply a twentieth-century problem. The Old Testament contains a number of accounts of barren women. Rachel cried out to her husband, Jacob, "Give me children or else I die." Her solution was to offer her maid, Bilhah, to Jacob in order that they might have children. The practice of using a surrogate mother appears to be having a resurgence in our own time. In some states, men with barren wives can donate sperm to a surrogate mother, generally through artificial insemination. She usually receives a fee of several thousand dollars for carrying the child to term and turning it over to the couple after it is born.

Another alternative to infertility, artificial insemination, is rapidly gaining acceptance. A fourteenth-century sheik, experimenting with horses, is thought to have been the first to impregnate livestock artificially. By now, the procedure has become a commonplace practice in animal husbandry. More than nine million cattle and nearly 150 million turkeys are artificially bred each year. Biologists think the method may save some endangered animal species from extinction. The number of human babies born through artificial insemination has been estimated at more than 20,000 a year.

Different women's reasons for resorting to artificial insemination can vary widely, but many seek it because their husbands have proved to be sterile. At one of the nearly two dozen sperm banks in the United States, thousands of semen samples are kept in storage, labeled according to each donor's physical, intellectual and genetic characteristics. All donors are carefully screened. One sperm bank in California is probably the most exclusive in the world: the only donors accepted are Nobel Award winners in science. Among sperm banks' other requirements, a donor's semen must be hardy enough to withstand freezing and thawing. It is often mixed with glycerol, a preservative, and frozen at temperatures as cold as −384° F. When sperm is frozen, it retains at least 60 percent of its potency for five years and sometimes longer. As an additional benefit, frozen sperm significantly reduces the frequency of birth defects and miscarriages.

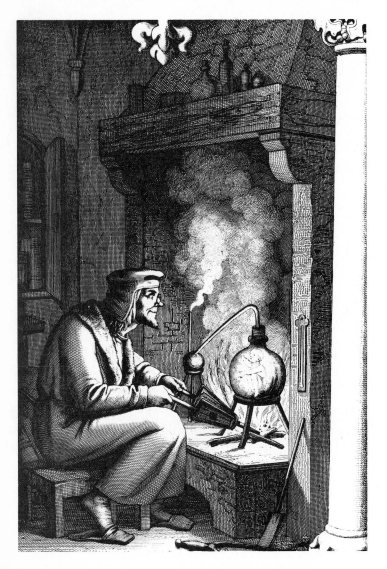

In a scene from Goethe's Faust, an alchemist intently fans his fire brighter with a bellows. The homunculus, a tiny man, that forms in the alembic is a fanciful precursor of modern science.

The procedures of artificial insemination are relatively simple. After a woman or a couple selects the desired characteristics of a donor, an ampule containing a little more than one cubic centimeter of semen is emptied into a syringe and injected into the woman's vagina. A rubber or plastic cap seals the vagina temporarily, preventing any semen from escaping. The procedure is painless, and some women even inseminate themselves at home. Artificial insemination by donor has made it possible for a single woman to bear a child without intercourse. Critics have added this technological innovation to the list of factors that they fear will undermine the family.

The controversy over artificial insemination is but a murmur compared to the clamor surrounding in vitro fertilization. Meaning "in glass," in vitro fertilization is known commonly — and mistakenly — as test-tube breeding. Fertilization in vitro means that a man's sperm and a woman's egg are united in a shallow glass or plastic Petri dish. When an embryo begins to form, it is placed in the woman's womb, providing the opportunity for a normal pregnancy. As more and more healthy children are born via the new procedure, it becomes clearer that in vitro fertilization ranks as one of the most dramatic biological achievements of our time.

Some people view in vitro fertilization as manipulative, a presumption of wisdom about the secrets of life that man is incapable of attaining. It is an old fear. Goethe's Faust tells of mysterious deeds done in a dark laboratory. Over a fire, one would-be creator heated an unholy substance in a glass vial and watched it slowly take form:

The glass vibrates with sweet and powerful tone;
It darkens, clears. . . .
And now in delicate shape is shown
A pretty manikin, moving, living, seeing!

The unnaturally conceived creature, a homunculus, or "little man," leads those assembled in the laboratory on a wondrous and terrible flight through night. It is the night of the witches' sabbath, Walpurgis Night, presided over by demons, specters and spirits of legend.

In vitro fertilization bears no resemblance to the macabre world of Faustian black magic. The

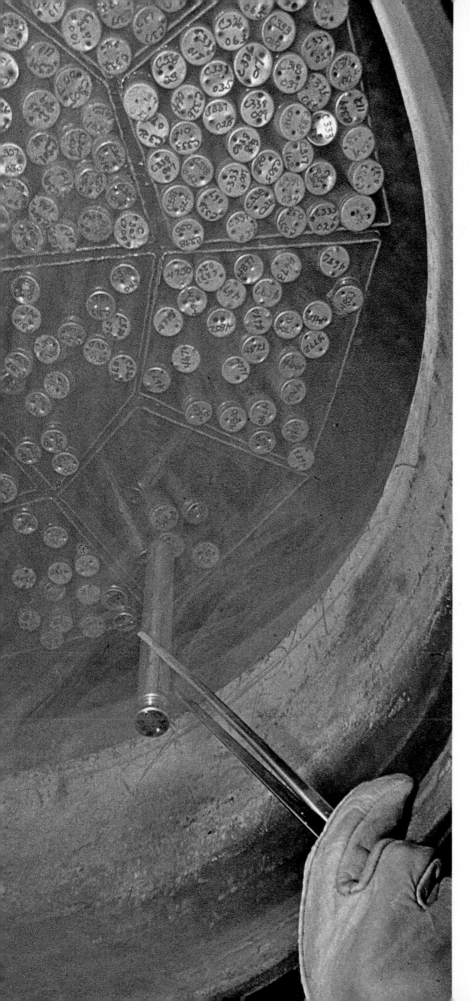

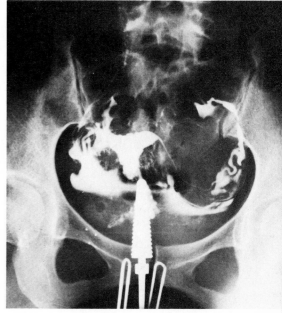

Plunged into a freezing vat of liquid nitrogen, ampules containing donated sperm, left, lie ready for use in a sperm bank. More than 20,000 births occur from artificial insemination in the United States each year. Techniques of artificial insemination have yielded unexpected benefits. The flexible cannula through which sperm is injected can also be used to open blockages of the uterine canal, above, giving some infertile women a chance to bear children.

idea of reproducing outside the body is ancient, as the Faust legend attests. As long ago as 1893, scientists began to experiment with external fertilization. In the 1950s, when rabbit eggs were fertilized outside the body, researchers began to turn their attention to higher mammals. Claims of human in vitro fertilization have been made since the 1940s, but the first confirmed instance occurred in England in 1969, under the direction of Robert Edwards, a Cambridge University physiologist, and Patrick Steptoe, an English gynecologist. Although the fertilized egg never left the laboratory dish, their report created a stir, and throughout the 1970s studies of human in vitro fertilization were done quietly and sometimes secretly. Finally, in 1978, Edwards and Steptoe announced that a woman was pregnant from the technique they had been perfecting for years. The woman was Lesley Brown, a thirty-year-old English housewife who had not conceived in nine years of marriage because of blocked Fallopian tubes. She became a celebrity on July 25, 1978, when she gave birth to a girl in a hospital in Oldham, a small city in northwestern England. Louise Brown was the first human baby conceived outside a mother's body.

The procedures that allow infertile women like Lesley Brown to have a child are the culmination of advances in medical equipment and in understanding the subtle physiological changes of pregnancy. One instrument that has proved indispensable to in vitro fertilization is the laparoscope, a device similar in principle to the periscope. It is a long metal tube about as thick as a pencil, containing a light and a tiny telescopic lens. Inserted through a small incision near the navel, the laparoscope permits a magnified view of a woman's ovaries, Fallopian tubes and other internal organs. By charting hormone levels in the woman's blood, physicians can predict almost the exact moment that an ovary will release an egg and witness it through a laparoscope. Hormones can be administered to ensure that an egg will be fully mature or to force the maturation of more than one ovum at a time. With a thin hollow needle inserted in the ovary's follicle, the place at which the egg will break free, the ovum is sucked out through a plastic tube and stored in a special culture that closely resembles conditions inside the womb. As one specialist in reproduction explains, "You don't want the eggs to suspect they are out of the body."

In the meantime, a sperm sample is obtained by masturbation and kept in a salt solution. The solution capacitates the sperm, meaning that it prepares the sperm for fertilization by removing chemical agents that prevent it from penetrating the egg. Inside the body, a woman's cervical secretions probably neutralize these inhibitors. The ovum, incubated for several hours after having been withdrawn from the ovary, is then placed in the solution with the sperm. Millions of tiny spermatozoa in the laboratory dish swim toward the egg, but only one will breach its outer layer. In about a day, the fertilized ovum, now called a zygote, begins to divide. After about two days, the zygote has formed between four and eight cells and is ready to be implanted in the woman. The nascent embryo is still so tiny that all work must be performed with the aid of a microscope.

Carefully drawing the embryo out of its dish into a cannula, or plastic tube, doctors insert it through the vagina into the uterus. If all goes well, the embryo will become embedded in the uterine wall and begin to develop normally. This delicate procedure has been the most difficult step in the complicated process of in vitro fertilization. Edwards and Steptoe achieved two pregnancies in their first seventy-nine attempts, but by 1982, the odds had improved to about one in ten. One peculiar observation noted by Edwards and Steptoe was that every successful implantation they performed had occurred at night. The reason is not known, but there is speculation that the body goes through different physiological stages at different times of the day.

America's In Vitro Baby

Now practiced in several countries, in vitro fertilization has become more than a medical curiosity. On December 28, 1981, Elizabeth Jordan Carr, America's first baby conceived in a laboratory dish, was born in Norfolk, Virginia. From complications incurred in previous pregnancies, the baby's mother, Judith Carr, had to have her Fallopian tubes removed. Still wanting a child,

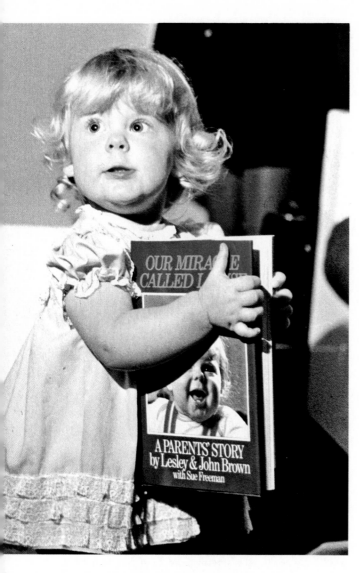

Louise Brown, the first "test-tube" baby, was born in Oldham England on July 25, 1978 as a result of in vitro fertilization. In the increasingly common procedure, a mature egg is drawn from the ovary of a woman whose diseased or injured Fallopian tubes block the egg's normal passage. Sperm from the husband is then mixed with the egg in a laboratory dish, and the newly developing embryo is implanted in the mother's womb.

she and her husband, Roger, went to the in vitro fertilization clinic of Howard and Georgeanna Jones at the Eastern Virginia Medical School. The Joneses, planning to retire from their distinguished careers in gynecology at Johns Hopkins University in Baltimore, arrived in Norfolk on the day Louise Brown was born in England. They opened a clinic early in 1980, but it took more than a year before they achieved the first pregnancy. Working with a team of specialists in reproduction, the Joneses have refined several techniques of in vitro fertilization, particularly in implanting the embryo in the mother.

At the time Elizabeth Carr was born, several other women treated at the Norfolk clinic were also pregnant. At least sixteen births had occurred in England and Australia through in vitro fertilization, with scores of other women expecting babies. Lesley Brown was pregnant with her second in vitro baby. Patients at the Joneses' clinic have expressed their relief and joy at having the opportunity to bear their own children. Howard Jones explains his own contribution humbly: "Any doctor who deals with infertility develops a very great reverence for life."

In vitro fertilization bypasses the Fallopian tubes altogether by taking a ripening egg directly from the ovary and mating it with sperm. Low tubal ovum transfer, a new fertility technique not yet used with human subjects, may offer an alternative to in vitro fertilization for women with blocked oviducts. In this new method, a maturing egg is removed from its follicle on the ovary, examined briefly and returned to the lower portion of the Fallopian tube, close to the opening into the uterus. With the egg moved past the obstruction in the oviduct, fertilization can take place through intercourse. The technique has been effective with experimental animals and may eventually become an option for infertile human couples as well.

For all the procreative abilities of mankind and the imaginative ways devised to bring about birth, many reproductive problems remain. In the United States, there are still 150,000 babies born with birth defects each year. The annual infant mortality rate in the United States, about 80,000 deaths, is higher than the rate in a dozen other

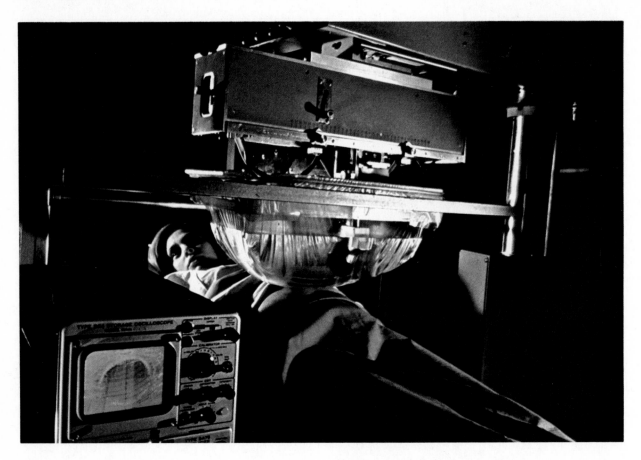

industrially developed countries. Every year, about 800 American women die during childbirth. The risk today is much lower than in decades past. In 1910, childbirth killed 17,000 women, a toll exceeded only by tuberculosis.

As new devices for assessing the health of a fetus have become commonplace, fetal monitoring, a whole new branch of obstetrics, has sprung up. Amniocentesis, first performed in 1919, has become a widely used method of detecting fetal abnormalities. Older mothers and other women considered at risk in bearing children with defects are particularly encouraged by doctors to undergo amniocentesis. Every fetus floats in a pool of amniotic fluid in its mother's womb. The fluid consists mostly of fetal urine but also contains liquids secreted through the skin and the respiratory tract of the fetus. In about the fifteenth week of pregnancy, a physician inserts a needle through the mother's abdominal wall to withdraw a small portion of the amniotic fluid. Doctors then assess the fetus's genetic health by examining cells in the fluid.

A new diagnostic tool, ultrasound, is rapidly gaining favor with physicians, especially obstetricians. Ultrasound relies on the same principle used in the sonar systems that detect submarines at sea. As practiced in fetal diagnosis, vibrations originate from a small crystal charged with an electric current. The crystal is usually in the end of a probe roughly the size of a hand-held microphone, which is placed on the mother's abdomen. High-frequency sound waves pass through the mother's body to the fetus and reflect to the sensitive probe as they meet the various organs of the fetus. These sound waves are converted to an electrical signal that registers as an image on a television screen. From her hospital bed, a pregnant woman can see the shape and movements of the baby inside her.

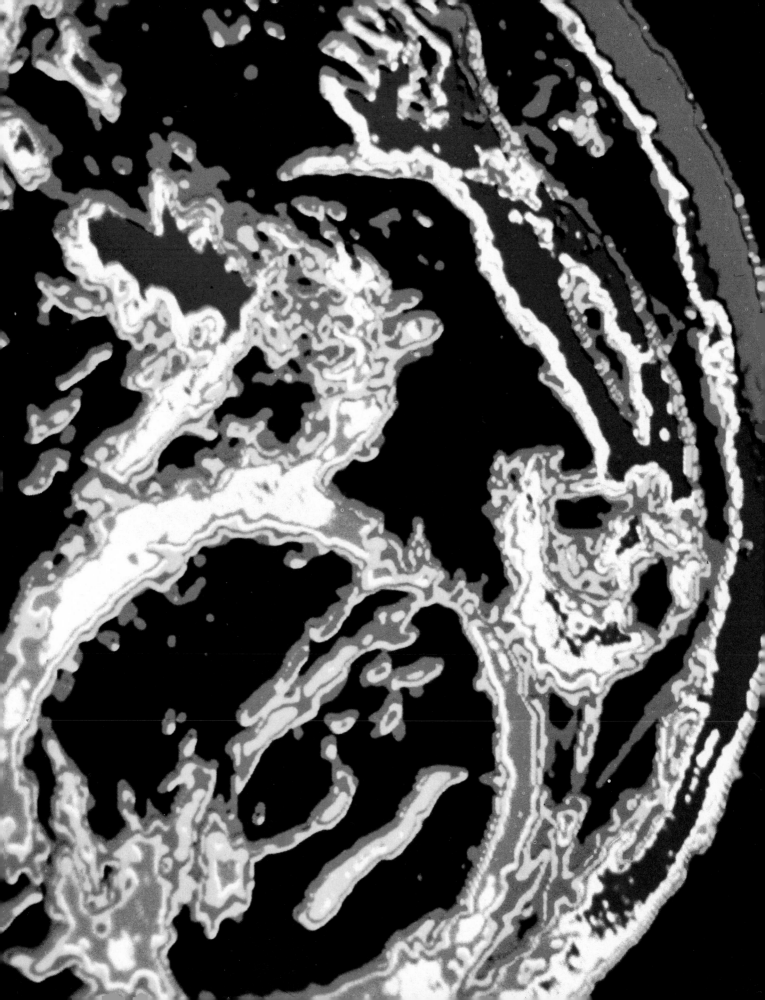

Michael Harrison and Mitchell Golbus

Treating the Youngest Patients

If doctors can identify a disease early, they stand a good chance of arresting it. But if it is noticed too late, even the most sophisticated medical techniques may do little good. Early diagnosis of fetal disorders can be especially frustrating because, as pediatric surgeon Michael Harrison says, "the patient isn't there." Harrison, obstetrician Mitchell Golbus and their colleagues at the University of California at San Francisco have found a way to help the most helpless patients. The doctors reach into the womb and operate on defective babies before they are born.

Before the advent of amniocentesis, ultrasound and other methods of assessing fetal health, prenatal surgery was inconceivable. But now, the hidden fetus has come into view. And by administering drugs that relax the uterus, the doctors can prevent premature labor contractions, perhaps the gravest risk in fetal surgery.

After Rosa Skinner, a forty-one-year-old mother of three, became pregnant in the fall of 1980, Golbus found through ultrasound that she was carrying twins. One twin appeared abnormal. Further tests revealed that the twins were fraternal — a boy and a girl — but that the boy had an

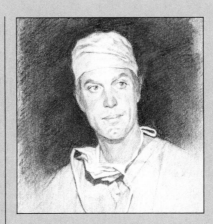

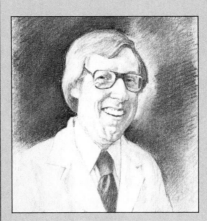

obstructed urinary tract. The first attempt to insert a catheter into the boy's bladder to drain urine failed. On Sunday, April 26, 1981, Harrison's surgical team operated again, guiding a redesigned catheter into place with the aid of ultrasound images. Later examinations showed that urine was draining properly. Two weeks later, the twins, Michael and Mary Skinner, were born.

Harrison and Golbus have reached another milestone in prenatal care by partially removing a fetus from its mother's womb and operating on urinary ducts leading from the kidneys. Their next goal is to repair fetal diaphragmatic hernia, a severe condition that prevents the lungs from developing. After that, they plan to tackle hydrocephalus, in which excess fluid can damage the brain. Golbus has also developed a new way of relieving malnutrition before birth. Nutrients are injected directly into the amniotic fluid, a source of fetal nourishment.

Fetal defects that yield to surgery are rare. Most are either too severe or can be dealt with after birth. Golbus says, "My biggest worry is that we might take a lesion that is fatal and correct it just enough that it is not fatal but is still incapacitating."

Although surgery is the most dramatic evidence of their work, Harrison and Golbus believe its greatest importance lies in a new understanding of fetal disease. Their goal, Harrison explains, is to "define the natural history of diseases which no one has even seen before." By pioneering surgery in the womb, they have provided new hope for the youngest patients of all.

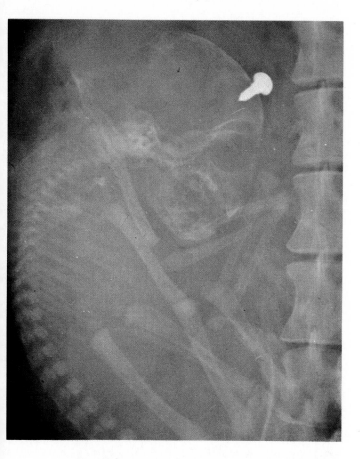

The techniques of ultrasound have become so refined that X-rays are now all but unnecessary in prenatal care. Not only does it render a lifelike image of the developing child, it also allows physicians to examine internal organs. Ultrasound can be used to diagnose fetal heart problems as early as the eighth week of pregnancy. It reveals soft tissues of the brain and provides an inner view of the chambers of the heart and the functioning of the heart's valves. Medical researchers have discovered that ultrasound can monitor eye movements during various stages of a fetus's growth. Abnormal movements are an early sign of developmental problems. Ultrasound is rapidly becoming a routine procedure in prenatal care. Not the least of its benefits, ultrasound harms neither mother nor fetus.

The fruits of medical technology have helped lower the infant mortality rate in the United States from 60 for every 1,000 births in 1930 to about a dozen per 1,000 births. With electronic devices, the baby's heart rate and the mother's uterine contractions can be measured throughout labor and delivery. Although premature babies weighing less than two pounds would not have survived only a few years ago, respirators and other advanced equipment can now bring many of them life. The babies are fed through tubes called catheters. But some parents and physicians have begun to question the value of some of these manmade interventions. Often, when a baby is premature or otherwise defective at birth, it can develop a series of related problems that could endanger its life or leave it seriously handicapped. Sometimes the treatment itself causes further complications. Complex ethical issues have increasingly entered the delivery room, compelling parents and doctors to weigh questions of survival against those of social usefulness and the expected quality of life.

Healing Before Birth

Surgery in the womb itself is a new choice for the parents of potentially defective children. For many years, researchers have been working with animals to develop a reliable way of preventing or relieving hydrocephalus, "water on the brain." Afflicting 4,200 newborn babies in the United States each year, hydrocephalus causes the ventricles of the brain, spaces filled with fluid, to expand grotesquely with liquid that would normally circulate through the brain and spinal cord. The pressure of the fluid prevents the brain cells from developing as they should and can lead to severe retardation, blindness, cerebral palsy, paralysis or death. After successful experiments on monkeys, surgeons first implanted a valve in the skull of a human fetus in 1981 to drain excess cerebrospinal fluid. If pressure inside the skull rises above the normal level, a needle-thin valve vents the excess fluid into the amniotic sac. In the studies on monkeys that cleared the path for human surgery, 80 percent of the monkeys survived and appeared healthy several months after birth. Only 10 percent of untreated monkeys were born alive, and all of them soon died.

Many fetal problems arise from the build-up of fluid in various parts of the body. In 1981,

Surgeons have entered the womb
to operate on a living fetus.
With delicate stitches, they opened
blocked urinary ducts, permitting
urine to pass into the surrounding
amniotic fluid.

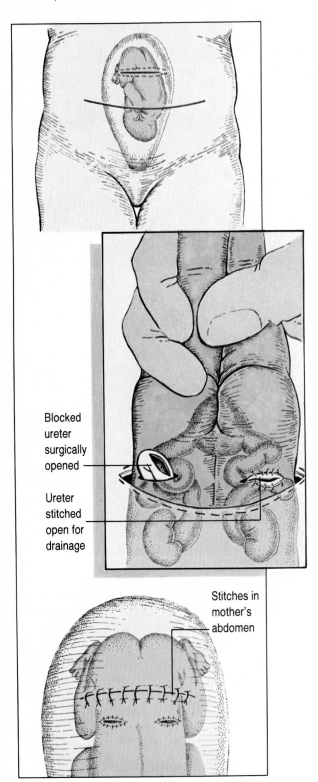

Blocked
ureter
surgically
opened

Ureter
stitched
open for
drainage

Stitches in
mother's
abdomen

doctors at the University of California at San Francisco learned from an ultrasound examination that a male fetus was developing ascites, an accumulation of fluid in the abdominal cavity. A team of physicians led by Michael Harrison and Mitchell Golbus determined that the cause of the problem was a blocked urinary tract. Untreated, the condition might have caused irreversible damage to the kidneys and lungs. The danger of attempting an operation to remedy the blockage was doubled because the fetus had a twin sister. Because Harrison and Roy Filly, another physician on the team, had previously operated on the bladders of fetal sheep and monkeys, they decided to go ahead with surgery. After implanting one catheter that did not stay in place, the doctors designed another with a flexible curve and inserted it in the fetus's bladder. The surgeons could not directly see the fetus during the operation and had to guide their movements by ultrasound images. The catheter discharged urine into the amniotic fluid and enabled the fetus to excrete without inadvertently endangering his life with the pressure of accumulating fluid. Both twins were healthy at birth, and with some corrective surgery, the boy is expected to recover and lead a normal life.

In a second operation, the San Francisco surgeons opened a woman's womb, partially removed the fetus to correct a kidney problem and returned it to the uterus. The mother was given a drug to prevent labor contractions during surgery. The fetus was delivered fourteen weeks after the operation, but died shortly after birth because its lungs had not developed adequately. Nevertheless, the work of the San Francisco team provides new hope for the unborn.

Another new surgical procedure developed in 1981 resulted in the deliberate abortion of one fetus but left its twin intact. Amniocentesis revealed that one twin was afflicted with Down's syndrome, a severe genetic disorder, and the parents planned to abort the pregnancy unless the normal baby could be saved. Using an ultrasound scanner to plot the location of the fetuses in the womb, surgeons withdrew the blood of the defective fetus. The other twin was born normally five months later. Because of the sensitive ethical

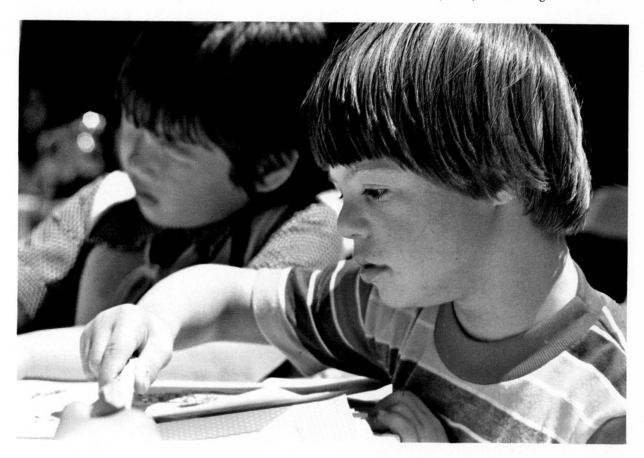

issues surrounding the operation, the hospital obtained a court order confirming the legality of the parents' decision.

Twins of a different sort — Siamese twins — have been the beneficiaries of surgery that separates their joined bodies, enabling them to lead ordinary lives. Originating from a single fertilized egg that did not completely divide to form identical twins, Siamese twins occur only about once in 100,000 births. Surgeons have separated perhaps two dozen sets of Siamese twins in extremely delicate operations made more difficult because the twins frequently share some organs. In March of 1982, surgeons at Baltimore's Johns Hopkins University separated Siamese twin sisters in a ten-hour operation. The single liver that the girls shared had to be divided, but liver tissue regenerates rapidly in infants. Doctors expect both twins to make complete recoveries after their unusual birth.

Because about 3 percent of all newborn babies have serious defects, surgery during pregnancy or just after birth may become more widespread in the future. Tens of thousands of infants who could once only be pitied may soon be offered the chance of full physical and mental health. Treatment of the youngest patients — infants and fetuses — is one of the fastest growing fields in medicine.

A smaller view of life, a microscopic view, has excited scientists and the public alike by unlocking doors that have hidden some of the secrets of early development. The study of embryology has brought to light the importance of the cell and how, in flurries of action, it is molded into living form. Cells connect with one another, scientists now believe, and learn from other cells around them. It appears that organs, limbs and functions develop, at least in part, because cells have the power of adaptation. As one part of the embryo

149

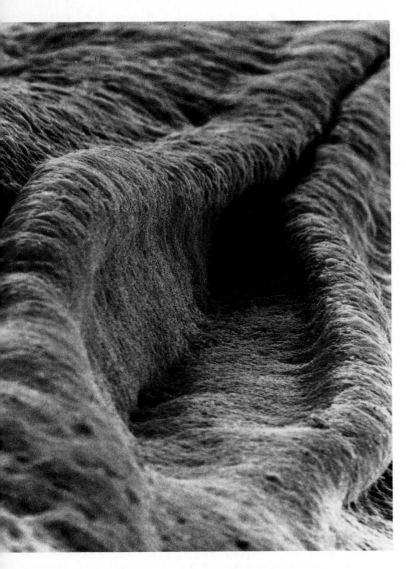

Magnified 600 times by a scanning electron microscope, the neural tube, a forerunner of the brain, spinal cord and backbone, begins to fuse. If the neural tube does not seal properly, serious birth defects can follow.

forms, other cells push ahead along biochemical paths to group with similar cells.

Knowledge of embryonic development has led to a new understanding of birth defects and disease. Scientists have observed that cancer cells behave in much the same manner as cells migrating in the embryo. Cancer cells proliferate and spread along the same routes that healthy embryonic cells follow. For this reason, some researchers think that if they can determine what causes an embryo's cells to split and move in the first place, they may be able to discover the source of cancer.

When something goes wrong with the cellular environment, the cells cannot respond correctly and may divide at the wrong time, too rapidly or not at all. Many birth defects seem to be caused in this way, as cells receive messages that disrupt their normal development. When surface antigens, molecules that relay messages from cell to cell, do not bind properly with hormones and other substances, cellular communication can break down and cause birth defects. Agents from outside the body are responsible for some of these abnormalities. Occasionally, though, the problem lies in defective genes, the tiny hereditary units that shape every individual's particular physical traits. A breakdown in the signals genes transmit can cause any of the more than 3,000 genetic disorders known.

Scientists have explored the roles of genes in an effort to decipher genetic codes that can carry disease or disfigurement. Some questions surrounding the influence of genes will probably never be completely resolved, but for now the soundest way of testing a fetus's genetic health is with amniocentesis. The most common genetic defect produces Down's syndrome, marked by mongoloid facial features, a stocky build and mental retardation. The disorder can be traced through analysis of the chromosomes, twisted threads of genes, in the amniotic fluid. Except for sperm and egg cells, which have half the normal chromosomes, human cells possess twenty-three pairs of chromosomes. Victims of Down's syndrome have an extra chromosome in the twenty-first position. For reasons not fully understood, older women are much more likely than younger women to bear children with Down's syndrome. Normally, the probability is roughly one in a thousand, but the chances increase to one in sixty between the ages of thirty-five and thirty-nine, and one in forty past the age of forty. A new blood test has been developed to identify women who might run the risk of having a child affected by Down's syndrome, before they become pregnant. Doctors have learned that a particular protein is found in the blood of mothers who have children with Down's syndrome that is not present in other women. The simple blood test is at least 90 percent accurate.

Amniocentesis can also reveal genetic disorders that affect certain groups of people more than others. Tay-Sachs disease is a rare disorder that produces deterioration of the nervous system and death in early childhood. Everyone is slightly at risk, but the disease is particularly prevalent among central or eastern European Jews, the Ashkenazi, occurring with a frequency of about one in 3,600 births. It is an inherited disease, and 3 to 4 percent of all Ashkenazi Jews are carriers.

Sickle cell anemia is a genetic blood disease that in its severest forms can lead to death. It is most common among blacks and some peoples of Mediterranean descent. A new method of fetal analysis, fetoscopy, can detect sickle cell anemia in fetuses, including the many cases that are missed by amniocentesis. Through a thin tube inserted into the fetal sac, a doctor can look directly at the fetus, much in the same way that fertility experts peer through a laparoscope to examine a woman's ovaries. Fetal blood samples can be drawn from the placenta, a membrane surrounding the fetus and lining the uterine wall. With a sample of scalp tissue no larger than the head of a pin, physicians can check for skin disease. Fetoscopy, though not widely practiced, is usually conducted between the fifteenth and twentieth weeks of pregnancy.

Screening Neural Defects

One of the saddest classes of genetic impairments is that of neural tube defects, affecting about one in 500 pregnancies in the United States, and about three times that number in Great Britain. In the first month of pregnancy, a roll of embry-

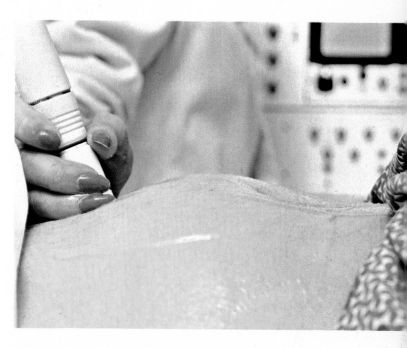

onic cells curls together, forming a tube. This neural tube eventually gives rise to the spinal cord and brain. If the tube does not seal completely, it can lead to spina bifida or anencephaly, two serious deformities. In spina bifida, the vertebrae do not form properly, leaving a hole through which the spinal cord protrudes. Babies born with this defect are usually paralyzed from the waist down and incapable of controlling their bowels and bladder. They often have hydrocephalus, as well, which commonly leaves them mentally retarded. With anencephaly, the other major neural tube defect, the brain and cranial vault do not develop at all. It is a mercy, perhaps, that most babies thus afflicted are stillborn or die soon after birth. The causes of these grave disorders are unknown. If a woman has had one child with a neural tube defect, she stands a 5 percent chance of having another.

A screening method recently devised can often spot neural tube defects by the presence of elevated levels of alphafetoprotein (AFP), a protein produced by the fetus, in the mother's blood. If a mother has high amounts of AFP, there is a distinct possibility that it leaked through a hole in the neural tube of the fetus. Ultrasound, amniocentesis and other tests can then be performed to

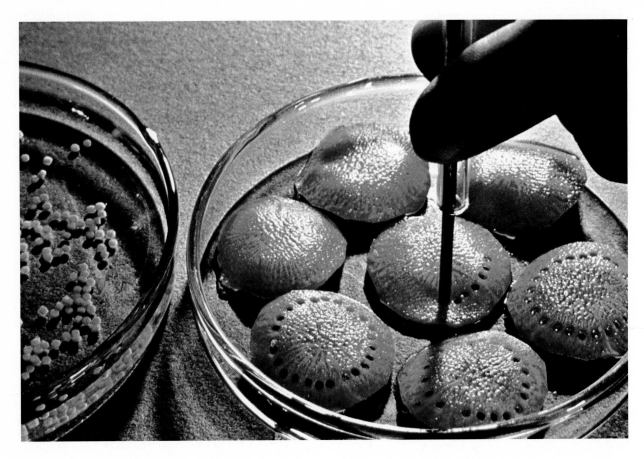

get a clearer idea of whether the fetus has a neural defect. This new test has caused some ethical concern because it sometimes forces parents to choose between abortion and the possibility of raising a child who may be either severely or mildly handicapped.

In the not-too-distant future, treatments that act on our genes may bring an end to some inherited diseases. Scientists have peered inside the gene at the spiral staircase of deoxyribonucleic acid, DNA, which carries instructions for the genes. They can replace sections of DNA, remove an individual gene from the DNA chain and duplicate it or even add a new gene to a growing embryo. As the roles of different genes become known, it will be only a matter of time before medicine begins to offer "gene therapy." In the laboratory, scientists have already developed techniques to create new forms of life by combining the DNA of different organisms.

Genes begin to act in the early stages of development after a sperm cell enters the egg. New DNA can be incorporated immediately after fertilization until the zygote has divided into four to eight cells. A biologist working with genes calls this "a privileged time" because the ovum chemically agrees to accept other genes, those from the sperm. Watching for this fleeting time, scientists have injected DNA from a rabbit into a mouse egg being fertilized by a sperm cell. Some of the offspring had the rabbit's gene as part of their genetic code. By this method, it may become an accepted practice to implant a gene in a human embryo to help a potential victim of diabetes, sickle cell anemia, muscular dystrophy or other debilitating disorders. With a desk-top device called a "gene machine," scientists can control chemical reactions to make synthetic copies of natural genes and splice them into the ribbon of DNA in a living cell. Alteration of living beings is

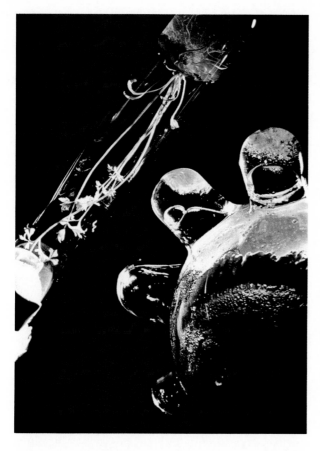

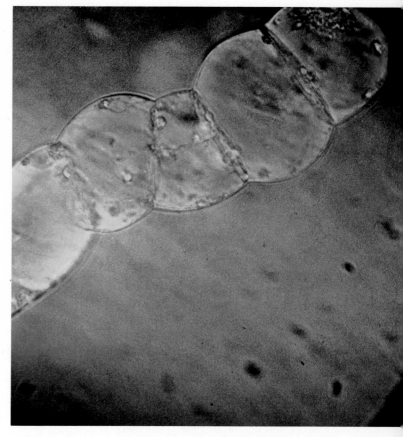

expected to have its widest use in agriculture. Plants could be genetically bred to resist disease, grow with little water or supply their own fertilizer. Livestock could be designed for their hardiness or ability to produce milk and meat.

With the power of genetic manipulation comes the possibility, and the fear, of cloning, the development of identical copies of a living organism. The idea is really not new; frogs were cloned from tadpole cells as early as 1952. The process is fairly common with some kinds of fish and with plants. Merely cutting a slip from a plant to start a new one in the garden is a form of cloning. In a 1979 experiment that is as close as science has come to cloning a mammal, researchers withdrew the nucleus from one cell of a four-day-old mouse embryo and transferred it into a fertilized egg from another mouse. The original sperm and egg nuclei about to fuse in the fertilized egg were removed. The new hybrid embryo, with genetic

Tiny plugs taken from carrot slices, opposite, can be used to clone the carrots, creating identical plants without sexual fertilization. Cells are specially treated to multiply as if they were growing from normal pollination, above left. A cell taken from almost any part of a mature carrot can produce another plant, like the one growing in the test tube, above right. Next to the test tube, a flask resembling a cow's udder separates individual cells when rotated.

Inside artificial wombs, fetal opossums receive milk and other nutrients from the hand of a scientist. Artificial wombs may become a tool in the struggle against fetal deaths and human infertility.

Like distant planets approaching eclipse, two mouse eggs join to form a single fertilized cell. The eggs combine without the presence of sperm, raising the possibility of asexual reproduction.

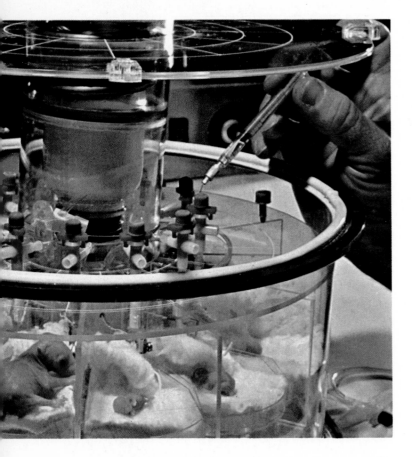

cannot differentiate into the countless functions that make up a human being. The only current evidence of human cloning is the replication of molecules of DNA.

Science has prudently moved in other directions, directions that have enhanced fertility and made life or parenthood possible where it was once a dream. Many of the newest techniques, such as freezing embryos or transferring multiple embryos from a prize mother to lesser stock, have wide application among animals but little or none among people. Other methods, though not in common practice, would surely raise questions about the legal and moral responsibilities of reproduction if they were. In laboratory glassware, scientists have combined two eggs and watched them join and divide as a normal embryo would, although no sperm touched either egg. Artificial wombs simulating the conditions of a woman's uterus may make it possible for premature babies to continue their development until the normal completion of their term. Although not yet possible, parents may someday be able to exercise a measure of control over their child's gender. By observing that male sperm cells, called Y sperm because they carry the male Y chromosome, swim faster than female X sperm, scientists may devise ways to collect disproportionate numbers of the speedy male sperm cells and, conversely, the slower female cells.

As the world grows more complex, as science reveals more about the secrets of living things, there is concern that man is turning a fragile, orderly universe into a nightmare. To many a mind come dark fantasies of a grim and repressive society like that of Aldous Huxley's *Brave New World,* where sperm and egg meet under microscopes and whole classes of people are bred anonymously for specific purposes, like so many bees. With these images in mind, it sometimes seems that fear is as natural as the change that causes it. Despite new customs that challenge established standards, there can be few things more hopeful than preparing for future generations and taking steps that will make their lives a little easier. Perhaps we have not given enough credit to our own common sense, our joy in life, our ways of using ingenuity wisely.

material from one developing mouse carried in another, was then placed in the uterus of a third mouse, a surrogate mother. The offspring were genetically identical to the original embryo. Many scientists hesitate to call this experiment an example of cloning because a new individual identical to another in a second generation was not formed. More accurately, the genetic contents of one embryo were born in another.

In the 1970s, there was a highly publicized story that an American millionaire had paid handsomely to have a clone of himself made. The tale has since been discredited as a hoax, but it raised an outcry among people who thought science had gone too far. More than any other field of reproductive technology, cloning has engendered implacable criticism from opponents who do not wish to see man try to create man in his own image. Many scientists believe human cloning is impossible because individual genes and cells

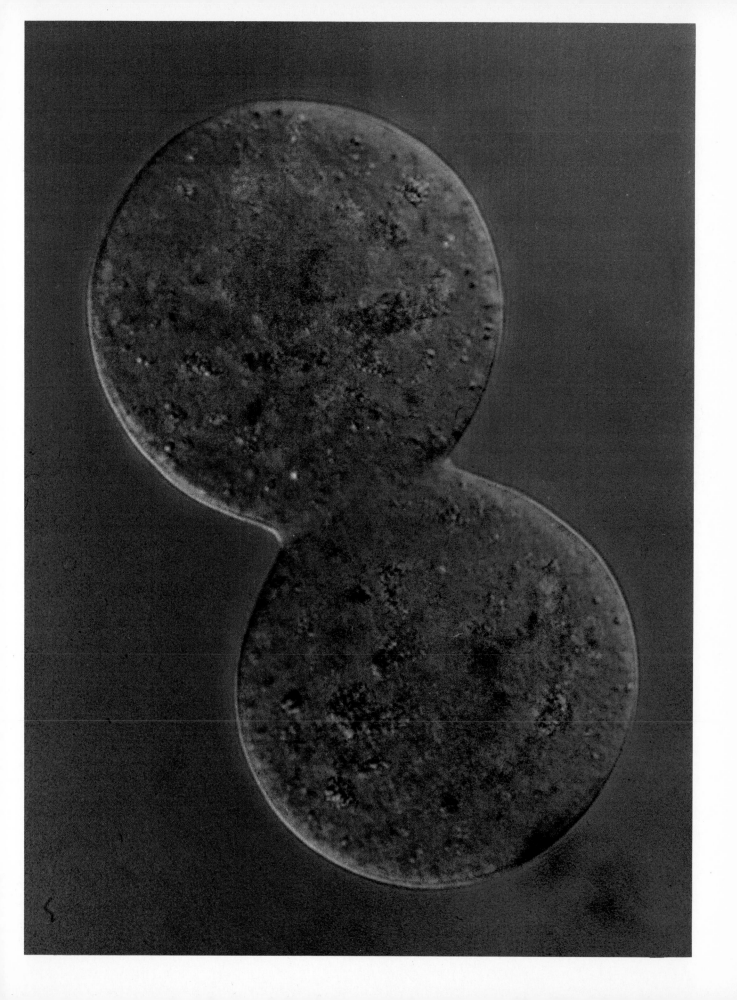

Glossary

abortion   the termination of pregnancy, by accident or design, before the fetus can survive outside the uterus.

acrosome   the forward end of the head of the sperm that releases enzymes to dissolve the surface of the ovum.

alphafetoprotein   AFP; a protein produced by the fetus which, detected in high levels in maternal blood, signals possible birth defects.

amniocentesis   a biochemical analysis of the amniotic fluid, withdrawn from the mother's abdomen, to assess fetal health and growth.

amnion   the innermost membrane enclosing the fetus.

amniotic fluid   the liquid surrounding the fetus.

analgesic   medication that reduces or eliminates the sensation of pain.

anencephaly   a deformity, usually fatal, in which the brain is missing and the skull is open.

anesthetic   an agent causing general unconsciousness or local insensitivity to pain.

animalcules   imaginary beings purported to exist within spermatozoa.

artificial insemination   the deliberate introduction of semen through the vagina to bring about pregnancy without sexual intercourse.

ascites   the excessive accumulation of serous fluid in the abdominal cavity.

autonomic nervous system   the part of the nervous system that regulates cardiac muscle activity and the work of smooth muscle and glands.

birth   parturition; the passage of the fetus from the uterus.

birthing chair   originally, a small stool on which a woman sat during labor and delivery; now made of fiber glass.

blastocyst   a stage in the development of the embryo marked by the differentiation of the cells into the trophoblast and embryoblast.

body stalk   the original link between the trophoblast and the embryoblast that joins with other fetal membranes to become the major part of the umbilical cord.

bonding   the establishment of a close relationship between child and parent; also the mating bond between individuals of the opposite sex.

breech birth   a baby delivered legs or buttocks first.

caesarean delivery   the birth of a fetus through an incision in the abdomen and uterus.

cannula   a slender tube for insertion into a duct or cavity.

castration   the removal of the testicles in men or the ovaries in women.

catecholamine   any one of several compounds containing epinephrine, norepinephrine and dopamine, believed to bring about labor.

caul   part of the membrane that surrounds a fetus, sometimes covering the head at delivery.

celibate   one who shuns marriage, generally by religious vows.

cervix   the neck of the uterus through which the fetus and menstrual fluids pass.

chancre   a hard ulcer, the first sign of syphilis.

changeling   a child surreptitiously swapped for another by spirits.

chastity   the abstention from sexual intercourse.

chloasma   the "mask of pregnancy"; pigmentation that creates a dark shadow cast over the nose and cheeks during pregnancy.

chorion   the outermost fetal membrane, enclosing the amnion, closest to the wall of the uterus.

chromosomes   threadlike elements within the nucleus of the cell that carry the genetic code.

circumcision   surgical excision of the foreskin of the penis.

climax   orgasm; the culmination of sex.

clitoris   a small oval of erectile tissue at the head of the vulva.

clomiphene citrate   Clomid; a synthetic analog of estrogen, the hormone that stimulates ovulation.

cloning   the production of identical copies of a living organism.

coition   coitus; sexual intercourse.

coitus interruptus   the withdrawal of the penis from the vagina before ejaculation of sperm.

colostrum   a secretion of serum and white blood cells from the breast before onset of lactation.

conception   the joining of sperm and ovum.

condom   a sheath of thin rubber that covers the penis during intercourse to prevent conception or transmittal of disease.

contraception   various methods of birth control that prevent conception.

copulation   the act of sexual intercourse.

corona glandis   the rounded border ringing the glans penis.

corpus luteum   a small yellow body formed at the ruptured follicle within the ovary during ovulation; it secretes hormones to maintain pregnancy until the placenta matures.

corticosteroids   synthetic steroid hormones.

couvade   the observance of specific rites and taboos, expressing symptoms of pregnancy, by the male to herald his imminent fatherhood.

couvade syndrome   sympathetic suffering by the male of the symptoms of pregnancy.

cytotrophoblast   the thin inner layer of the trophoblast.

Demerol   trade name of meperidine hydrochloride, a synthetic pain reliever.

demography   the study of the growth, change and structure of populations.

deoxyribonucleic acid   DNA; a complex molecule in cells that carries genetic information.

diaphragm   a flexible disk fitted over the cervix, barring the passage of semen to prevent conception.

diethylstilbestrol   DES; a synthetic estrogen.

dominant gene   a gene that produces the same characteristics when paired with either an identical or dissimilar gene.

Down's syndrome   mongolism; an abnormality caused by an extra chromosome; distinguished by mental retardation and changed physical appearance.

ectoderm   the outermost layer of cells in the developing embryo.

ectopic pregnancy   a pregnancy in which the zygote implants itself outside the uterus.

ejaculation   the expulsion of semen from the penis.

embryo   the human organism between its second and eighth weeks of development.

embryo transfer   in animal husbandry, the transfer of an embryo from one mother to another.

embryoblast   the inner cell mass of the blastocyst from which the embryo forms.

embryology   the science of the origins and development of individual living organisms.

embryonic disk   a structure in the stage of the development of the embryo marked by the formation of ectoderm, mesoderm and endoderm.

emission   the involuntary discharge of semen into the urethra.

endoderm   the innermost layer of cells in the developing embryo.

endometrium   the innermost lining of the uterus.

epididymis   the twisted duct lying behind and leading from each testicle.

epidural   a form of regional anesthesia administered in the mother's lower back to ease the pain of childbirth.

epinephrine   adrenalin; a hormone that stimulates the sympathetic nervous system to control blood pressure, increase metabolism and induce uterine contractions.

erection   the swelling stiffness of the penis in men and the clitoris in women during sexual excitement.

estrogen   a female sex hormone responsible for secondary sex characteristics, the menstrual cycle and pregnancy.

estrus   the cyclical period of sexual activity in mammals, except for some primates; the state of being in heat.

Fallopian tube   oviduct; the tube leading from the ovary to the uterus.

fertility   the capability to reproduce.

fertility drug   a hormone, either natural or synthetic, administered to induce ovulation.

fertilization   conception; the union of sperm and ovum.

fetal alcohol syndrome   FAS; those symptoms common among offspring of mothers who drink heavily during pregnancy.

fetoscopy   direct visual observation of the fetus through a tube to monitor growth and development.

fetus   the human organism between the ninth week of its development and its birth.

fibrinolysin   an enzyme that prevents clotting of the blood, released during menstruation.

follicle   a round structure at the ovary consisting of the oocyte and the cells surrounding it.

follicle-stimulating hormone   FSH; a hormone released by the pituitary gland that stimulates the growth of the follicle and spermatogenesis.

forceps   an instrument that grasps a baby's head, sometimes used to ease a difficult delivery.

foreskin   prepuce; loose folds of skin shrouding the end of the penis or hooding the clitoris.

frigidity   a lack of libido or interest in sex, referring chiefly to women.

genes   the smallest factor responsible for passing inherited characteristics from parents to offspring.

genetics   the science dealing with the passing of physical and chemical characteristics from parents to offspring and the impact of the environment on genes and genetic expression.

genitals   the organs of reproduction.

gestational diabetes   a form of diabetes peculiar to pregnancy.

glans penis   the smooth, domed tip of the penis.

glycerol   a clear, colorless, syrupy fluid; a product formed by the hydrolysis of fat.

gonadotropin-releasing factor   a substance causing the pituitary gland to release luteinizing hormone (LH) and follicle-stimulating hormone (FSH).

gonorrhea   a sexually transmitted disease caused by bacteria that invade the urogenital tract.

gynecology   the branch of medicine treating diseases peculiar to females, especially of the genital, urinary and rectal organs.

herpes   a group of viruses causing a number of diseases, among them chicken pox, shingles and genital herpes.

herpes simplex II   a sexually transmitted virus causing genital lesions and ulcers for which there is no cure.

homosexuality   sexual desire for and activity with members of one's own sex.

human chorionic gonadotropin   HCG; a hormone produced by the chorionic villi, triggering the release of estrogen and progesterone.

human menopausal gonadotropin   a fertility drug; a hormone taken from the urine of postmenopausal women to promote ovulation.

Huntington's chorea   a rare hereditary disorder of the nervous system causing involuntary movement and mental disarray.

hyaluronic acid   an extracellular substance that cements cells together and retains water in tissues between cells.

hyaluronidase   an enzyme released by the acrosome that dissolves the surface of the ovum.

hydrocephalus   a congenital abnormality marked by the accumulation of excess fluid in the skull.

hymen   a membrane wholly or partially occluding the vaginal opening.

implantation   the process by which the blastocyst embeds itself in the wall of the uterus.

impotence   the failure to maintain an erection and so perform sexual intercourse.

infanticide   the killing of newborn infants, generally the weak, ill or unwanted.

infant mortality rate   the number of annual deaths of infants under one year of age usually per 1,000 live births.

infertility   sterility, barrenness; the inability to reproduce sexually.

intrauterine device   IUD; a device of plastic or metal placed in the uterus as a means of birth control.

in vitro fertilization   the fertilization of an ovum by a sperm under laboratory conditions.

labia majora   the twin folds of skin covered with pubic hair around the vaginal opening.

labia minora   two thin folds of skin lying inside the labia majora.

labor   the set of processes which expels the fetus from the uterus.

laparoscopy   visual examination of the interior of the abdomen, particularly of a woman's ovaries, through a telescopic device passed through the abdominal wall.

Lesch-Nyhan syndrome   an inherited disorder of males characterized by men-tal retardation, spastic cerebral palsy and bizarre behavior, even self-mutilation.

Leydig cells   cells of the testicles that produce the male hormone testosterone.

low tubal ovum transfer   the removal of a maturing ovum from the ovary and its placement in the lower portion of the Fallopian tube.

luteinizing hormone   LH; a hormone produced by the pituitary gland.

mammary gland   the gland in the female breast that secretes milk.

mammography   radiographic examination of the breast.

mastectomy   surgical removal of the breast.

masturbation   exciting the genitalia, usually to orgasm, by means other than sexual intercourse.

menopause   "change of life"; the time when menstruation ceases, usually between the ages of forty-five and fifty.

menstruation   menses; the periodic discharge of bloody fluid from the uterus through the vagina, occurring between puberty and menopause.

mesoderm   the middle layer of cells in the developing embryo.

midwife   a person skilled in the art of assisting in childbirth.

miscarriage   the spontaneous loss of pregnancy before the fetus can survive outside the womb.

mons pubis   a fleshy pad of fatty tissue covering the pubic bone in females.

mons veneris   the mons pubis.

natural selection   the Darwinian principle that individuals with characteristics best suited to survival in a particular environment become a greater proportion of their species within that environment with each generation.

neural tube   the longitudinal tube within the embryo from which the nervous system develops.

norepinephrine   noradrenalin; a hormone that functions like epinephrine.

notochord   a tube of cells joined in the embryo foreshadowing the spine.

obstetrics   the branch of medicine dealing with the care of women during pregnancy, at childbirth and after delivery.

oocyte   a descendant of an oogonium that divides to produce an ovum.

oogenesis   the process by which the ovum reaches maturity.

oogonium   a descendant of immature sex cells that give rise to oocytes.

ovary   one of a pair of glands in the female, on each side of the pelvic cavity, that produces ova and hormones.

ovulation   the periodic production and discharge of an ovum by the ovary.

ovum   egg; the female reproductive cell.

oxytocin   the hormone produced by the pituitary gland that stimulates contractions of the uterus and release of milk at the breasts.

Pap test   a microscopic examination of scrapings from the cervix that reveals premalignant or malignant cells.

penis   the male organ for urination and copulation.

pessary   a device put inside the vagina to support the uterus or to prevent conception.

pheromone   a chemical secreted by an animal that attracts the opposite sex of the same species.

phocomelia   a physical deformity marked by the failure of limbs to develop fully.

pica   cravings for bizarre or unusual substances sometimes experienced during pregnancy.

pituitary gland   hypophysis; a small, oval endocrine gland lodged at the base of the brain that affects other endocrine glands.

placenta   a temporary organ which exchanges nutrients and wastes between mother and fetus and produces hormones needed to maintain pregnancy.

polar body   a small body cast off by the primary oocyte as it matures.

preeclampsia-eclampsia   hypertension and edema brought about by pregnancy; a disorder occurring after the twentieth week of gestation.

premature birth   a birth occurring before the fetus completes thirty-seven weeks of gestation.

premenstrual syndrome   PMS; physical discomfort and emotional tension preceding the onset of menstruation.

primitive streak   a thick, opaque groove in the ectoderm that accompanies the emergence of the mesoderm and notochord.

primordia   the forerunners of organs or other structures in the embryo.

progesterone   a hormone produced by the corpus luteum and placenta that readies the endometrium for implantation, breasts for lactation and maintains the pregnancy.

prolactin   lactogenic hormone; the hormone produced by the pituitary gland that encourages growth of breast tissue and lactation.

prostaglandins   PG; fatty acid derivatives; substances widespread in body tissues having many functions in reproduction.

prostate   a gland surrounding the urethra at the neck of the bladder in men.

puberty   the stage when an individual becomes capable of reproduction.

quickening   the moment the mother first senses fetal movement.

recessive gene   a gene that does not produce a visible feature when paired with a dissimilar gene.

recombinant DNA   DNA artificially drawn from one species, combined with DNA from the same or a different species and transplanted to the original or another species.

relaxin   a hormone that inhibits uterine contractions, possibly helping to prevent premature labor; it may also soften the cervix to make birth easier.

ritodrine hydrochloride   a smooth muscle relaxant.

rubella   German measles; a viral disease hazardous to embryonic development.

scrotum   the soft pouch holding the testicles and accessory organs.

secondary oocyte   a stage in the maturation of the ovum.

semen   a white viscous secretion of the male reproductive organs that carries sperm.

seminiferous tubules   the small tubes of the testicles that produce sperm.

Sertoli cells   cells in the seminiferous tubules that nurture developing sperm.

sexual selection   the companion hypothesis to natural selection which holds that characteristics that best equip males for courtship and combat become preferred in their progeny.

Siamese twins   twins born with their bodies joined together.

sickle cell anemia   an inherited form of anemia marked by the presence of deformed, oxygen-poor red blood cells.

somites   blocks of mesoderm from which skeletal, muscle and some skin tissue grows.

sperm   the male reproductive cell.

sperm bank   a depository of sperm for use in artificial insemination.

spermatids   the penultimate stage in the development of sperm.

spermatogenesis   the process by which sperm develops.

spermatogonium   the primordial sperm.

spermatozoon   sperm; the mature male reproductive cell.

spina bifida   a congenital abnormality characterized by the failure of the backbone to fuse.

spirochetes   slender, twisted microorganisms, many of which cause diseases, among them syphilis.

surrogate mother   a woman who agrees to bear a child for another.

syncytiotrophoblast   the outer layer of the trophoblast that invades the endometrium.

syphilis   a sexually transmitted disease that progresses from chancres to ulcers and finally to general paresis.

Tay-Sachs disease   the infantile form of a group of diseases marked by progressive blindness, mental deterioration and loss of motor control, ending in death by the age of three.

testicles   the two reproductive glands that produce male reproductive cells and testosterone.

testosterone   the principal steroid hormone produced in men, responsible for secondary sex characteristics.

thalidomide   a chemical used in Europe as a sedative until found to cause phocomelia in fetuses.

trophoblast   the blastocyst's outermost layer which produces the placenta.

Turner's syndrome   a sexual aberration caused by a missing X chromosome in females.

ultrasound   the use of high-frequency sound waves to monitor fetal growth and development.

umbilical cord   the tube joining the placenta and the fetus.

uterus   the womb; a hollow, muscular organ where the fetus is implanted, sheltered and nurtured.

vagina   the passageway between the uterus and the vulva.

varicocele   a condition of the testicle in which enlargement of veins can inhibit the production of sperm, causing infertility.

vas deferens   the excretory duct of each testicle that conveys sperm.

vasectomy   the surgical sterilization of men by incising or tying off the vasa deferentia, possibly reversible, usually permanent.

vulva   the external genitalia of the female.

zygote   the fertilized ovum.

Illustration Credits

Replenishing Our Kind
6, Euro Color Library.

From Genesis to Genetics
8, *The Kiss* by Gustav Klimt, Osterreichisches Museum für Angewandte Kunst, Vienna, by permission of Verlag Galerie Welz Salzburg. 10, The Bettmann Archive. 11, M. Philip Kahl/Photo Researchers, Inc. 12, (top) Douglas Masonowicz, Gallery of Prehistoric Art, New York City (bottom) from *The Mystery of Sex*; English translation © 1960, Elek Books Ltd.; published by arrangement with Lyle Stuart. 13, Douglas Masonowicz, Gallery of Prehistoric Art, New York City. 14-17, The Bettmann Archive. 18, Sonia Halliday Photographs. 18-19, *Birth of Venus* by Botticelli, SCALA/Editorial Photo Archives. 20, **Thomas B. Allen.** 21, Kongelige Bibliothek, Copenhagen. 22 and 23, Royal Library, Windsor Castle; reproduced by gracious permission of Her Royal Majesty Queen Elizabeth II. 24-26, Historical Collections, College of Physicians of Philadelphia. 27, Smithsonian Institution Libraries. 29, (left) The Bettmann Archive (right) Ann Ronan Picture Library. 30, Jack Couffer/Bruce Coleman, Inc. 31, Bruce Coleman/Bruce Coleman, Inc. 32, *Month of April* by Francesco del Cossa, SCALA/Editorial Photo Archives. 33, Courtesy of the Freer Gallery of Art, Smithsonian Institution. 34, The Mansell Collection, Ltd. 35, From the *Wolf-Man* by the Wolf-Man, edited by Muruel Gardiner; © 1971, Basic Books, Inc., used by permission. 36, © Arnold Newman. 37, Edward Quinn/Gamma. 38, Jan Halaska/Photo Researchers, Inc. 39, Drawing by Drucker; © 1978, The New Yorker, Inc.

The Seeds of Life
40, *God Admonishing Adam and Eve,* Mosaic from Monreal, SCALA/Editorial Photo Archives. 42, *The Circumcision of Christ* by Giovanni Bellini, The Granger Collection, New York. 43, **Mark Seidler.** 44, **Scott Barrows** (photo inset) from *Tissues and Organs: A Text-Atlas of Scanning Electron Microscopy* by Richard G. Kessel and Randy H. Kardon; © 1979, W. H. Freeman & Co. 45, © London Scientific Fotos. 46, (left) **Karen Karlsson** (right) Arthur M. Siegelman/FPG. 49, **Mark Seidler.** 50, Francis Countway Medical Library. 51, (left) The Granger Collection, New York (right) Manfred Kage/Peter Arnold, Inc. 52, (left) **Karen Karlsson.** 52 and 53, **Scott Barrows.** 54, Lennart Nilsson from his book *Behold Man*, published in the U. S. by Little, Brown & Co., Boston. 56 and 57, Phillip A. Harrington/Peter Arnold, Inc. 58, Howard Sochurek/Woodfin Camp & Assoc. 59, **Thomas B. Allen.** 60, The Bettmann Archive. 61,

Courtesy of the Wellcome Trustees. 62, **George V. Kelvin**/Science Graphics. 63, Eric Grave/Photo Researchers, Inc. 65, **Mark Seidler.** 66, (left) "Sea urchin sperm-egg interactions studied with the scanning electron microscope," M. Tegner and D. Epel, *Science,* Vol. 179, pp. 685-688, Fig. 2c, Feb. 16, 1973, © 1973 by the American Association for the Advancement of Science (right) sea urchin (*Arabacia punctulata*) sperm-egg interaction, Drs. D. W. Fawcett and E. Anderson, Harvard Medical School. 67, Dr. Mia Tegner, Scripps Institution of Oceanography, University of California, San Diego. 68, *Family Kaiser Maximiliaus I* by B. Strigel, Kunsthistorisches Museum, Vienna. 69, The Bettmann Archive.

A Sudden Quickening
70, *Maternité* by Marc Chagall, Stedelijk Museum, Amsterdam. 73, **Carol Donner.** 74, 76 and 77, Lennart Nilsson from his book *A Child Is Born*, published in the U. S. by Dell Publishing Co., Inc., New York. 78, Joe Baker/FPG. 79, (left) © London Scientific Fotos. 79, (right) and 81, Lennart Nilsson from his book *A Child Is Born*, published in the U. S. by Dell Publishing Co., Inc., New York. 82, Yale Medical Library, New Haven, CT. 83, A. R. Williams, Charing Cross Hospital, London Scientific Fotos. 84, © 1982, Erika Stone. 85, National Library of Medicine. Foldout (left) Lennart Nilsson from his book *A Child Is Born*, published in the U. S. by Dell Publishing Co., Inc., New York (right) Lennart Nilsson from his book *Behold Man*, published in the U. S. by Little, Brown & Co., Boston (inside) **Christine D. Young.** 87, National Library of Medicine. 89, (top) Leonard McCombe, *Life* © 1969, Time Inc. (bottom) acknowledgment is made to the C. V. Mosby Co. for permission to reprint published material appearing in the *American Journal of Obstetrics and Gynecology*.

Of Woman Born
90, *Le Berceau* by Berthe Morisot, The Granger Collection, New York. 92, The Granger Collection, New York. 93 and 94, The Bettmann Archive. 95, James Schweiker/*The Saturday Evening Post,* © 1982. 96-97, **Susan Hilfer.** 97, (right) Eve Arnold/Magnum. 98, The Mansell Collection Ltd. 99, Uwe Ahrens/*Eltern.* 100, David Hurn/Magnum. 101, © London Scientific Fotos. 103, Collection of G. E. Mestler, Downstate Medical Center, Brooklyn. 104, **Pat Kenny.** 105, Mariette Pathy Allen. 107, David A. Kliot, M. D. 108, Skip Brown. 109, Karen Keeny/Woodfin Camp, Inc. 110, Uwe Ahrens/*Eltern.* 111, (top) *Madonna and Child* by Andrea Mantegna, Samuel H. Kress Collection, National Gallery of Art, Washington (bottom) **Joyce**

Hurwitz. 112, (top) © 1982, Mickey Pfleger (bottom) Walter Salinger, reproduced by permission of Anthony DeCasper. 113, Camilla Smith/Rainbow.

An Elusive Balance
114, *Noah Loading the Animals Two by Two,* Swiss Panel, 1682, in the Church of St. Michael and Our Lady at Wragby, Yorkshire, Sonia Halliday and Laura Lushington. 116, © Van Bucher/Photo Researchers, Inc. (chart inset) **Jennifer Arnold.** 117, *Mese di Luglio,* from fresco in Castello del Buonconsiglio, Trento, SCALA/Editorial Photo Archives. 118, The Mary Evans Picture Library. 119, The Granger Collection, New York. 120, **Thomas B. Allen.** 121, The Granger Collection, New York. 122, BBC Hulton Picture Library. 123, The Bettmann Archive. 124, Paolo Koch/Photo Researchers, Inc. 125, The Granger Collection, New York. 126, © Ted Horowitz/Intermarco Advertising, Inc., NY and Ansell, Inc. NJ, all rights reserved. 127, **Graziella Becker.** 128, (both) Robert Noonan/Photo Researchers, Inc. 129, **Thomas B. Allen.** 130, Printed by permission of Planned Parenthood Federation of America, Inc., New York. 131, Martin Rogers. 132, Paolo Koch/Photo Researchers, Inc. 133, Dean Brown/Nancy Palmer Photo Agency, Inc.

Braving the New World
134, Fritz Goro, *Life* © 1965, Time Inc. 137, **Thomas B. Allen.** 138, Historical Picture Service, Chicago. 139, Craig W. Laube & Jonathan D. Robinson, Akron, OH. 140, The Bettmann Archive. 141, (left) John Marmaras/Woodfin Camp & Assoc. (right) Tomonobu Ikeda, Japan. 143, Lester Sloan/*Newsweek.* 144, Fritz Goro, *Life* © 1965, Time Inc. 145, Howard Sochurek/Woodfin Camp & Assoc. 146, **Thomas B. Allen.** 147, Pregnancy Research Branch, National Institute of Child Health and Human Development. 148, **Joyce Hurwitz.** 149, Richard Hutchings/Photo Researchers, Inc. 150, John-Paul Revel, California Institute of Technology. 151, Kenneth Garrett/Woodfin Camp, Inc. 152-154, Fritz Goro, *Life* © 1965, Time Inc. 155, © Fritz Goro, courtesy of Life Picture Service.

160

Index

Page numbers in bold type indicate location of illustrations.

162

virginity, 19, 48, 50
virus, 85
vitamin, 80, 85
  E, 57
vulva, 13

W
waste, 80
water, 41, 80
  immersion in, 10

Watson, James, 29
Wilde, Friedrich Adolph, 126
Wilson, Edward O., 33-34
wind, 10, 18
Wolf Man, 35
Woman Rebel, 128
womb, 7, 13, 17, 18, 19, 20, 22, 24, 48, 53, 64-65, 80, 81-82, 93, 94, 98, 99, 100, 101, 102, 103, 107, 127, 131, 135, 142, 143, 144, 146, 147, 148, 154, *see also* uterus

X
Xenophon, 47
X-ray, 29, 58, 102, 147

Y
yin and yang, 13
yolk sac, 50, *fold-out*
Yolles, Stanley F., 38-39

Z
Zeus, 19
zygote, 71-72, 142, 152